Fundamentals of Clinical Ophthalmology

Plastic and Orbital Surgery

Fundamentals of Clinical Ophthalmology series

Glaucoma
Edited by Roger Hitchings

Neuro-ophthalmology
Edited by James Acheson and Paul Riordan-Eva

Paediatric Ophthalmology
Edited by Anthony Moore

Scleritis
Edited by Peter McCluskey

Uveitis
Edited by Susan Lightman and Hamish Towler

Forthcoming:

Cataract Surgery
Edited by David Garty

Cornea
Edited by Douglas Coster

Strabismus
Edited by Frank Billson

Fundamentals of Clinical Ophthalmology

Plastic and Orbital Surgery

Edited by

Richard Collin
Consultant Ophthalmic Surgeon,
Moorfields Eye Hospital,
London, UK

and

Geoffrey Rose
Consultant Ophthalmic Surgeon,
Moorfields Eye Hospital,
London, UK

Series Editor
Susan Lightman
Professor of Clinical Ophthalmology,
Institute of Ophthalmology/Moorfields Eye
Hospital, London, UK

© BMJ Books 2001
BMJ Books is an imprint of the BMJ Publishing Group

First published in 2001
by BMJ Books, BMA House, Tavistock Square,
London WC1H 9JR

www.bmjbooks.com

British Library Cataloguing in Publication Data

A catalogue record for this book is available from the British Library

ISBN 0-7279-1475-8

Typeset by FiSH Books
Printed in Malaysia by Times Offset

Contents

Contributors

Michèle Beaconsfield
Consultant Ophthalmic Surgeon, Moorfields Eye Hospital, London, UK

Richard N Downes
Consultant Ophthalmic Surgeon, General Hospital, St Helier, Jersey, CI

Carole A Jones
Consultant Ophthalmic Surgeon, Kent County Ophthalmic and Aural Hospital, Maidstone, UK

Ewan G Kemp
Consultant Ophthalmologist, Gartnavel General Hospital, Glasgow, UK

Carol Lane
Consultant Ophthalmic Surgeon, University Hospital of Wales, Cardiff, UK

Brian Leatherbarrow
Consultant Ophthalmic, Oculoplastic and Orbital Surgeon, Manchester Royal Eye Hospital, Manchester, UK

Christopher J McLean
Consultant Ophthalmic Surgeon, Royal Surrey County Hospital, Guildford, UK

Alan A McNab
Consultant Ophthalmic Surgeon, Royal Victorian Eye and Ear Hospital, The Royal Melbourne Hospital and the Royal Children's Hospital, Melbourne, Australia

Ruth Manners
Consultant Ophthalmic Surgeon, Southampton General Hospital, Southampton, UK

Brett O'Donnell
Consultant Ophthalmic Surgeon, Royal North Shore Hospital and St Vincent's Hospital, Sydney, Australia

Jane M Olver
Consultant Ophthalmic Surgeon, The Western Eye Hospital, London, UK

John Pitts
Consultant Ophthalmologist, Barts and the London NHS Trust, London, UK

Cornelius René
Consultant Ophthalmic Surgeon, Addenbrooke's Hospital, Cambridge, UK

Fiona Robinson
Consultant Ophthalmologist, King's College Hospital, London, UK

Timothy J Sullivan
Clinical Associate Professor and Head, Department of Ophthalmology, Royal Brisbane Hospital, Brisbane, Australia

Anthony G Tyers
Consultant Ophthalmologist, Salisbury District Hospital, Salisbury, UK

Michael J Wearne
Consultant Ophthalmic Surgeon, Eastbourne District Hospital, Eastbourne, UK

Preface to the

Fundamentals of Clinical Ophthalmology series

This book is part of a series of ophthalmic monographs, written for ophthalmologists in training and general ophthalmologists wishing to update their knowledge in specialised areas. The emphasis of each is to combine clinical experience with the current knowledge of the underlying disease processes.

Each monograph provides an up to date, very clinical and practical approach to the subject so that the reader can readily use the information in everyday clinical practice. There are excellent illustrations throughout each text in order to make it easier to relate the subject matter to the patient.

The inspiration for the series came from the growth in communication and training opportunities for ophthalmologists all over the world and a desire to provide clinical books that we can all use. This aim is well reflected in the international panels of contributors who have so generously contributed their time and expertise.

Susan Lightman

Preface

This book covers the whole field of eyelid, lacrimal, orbital and socket surgery. As part of the series of ophthalmic monographs it is written for ophthalmologists in training and general ophthalmologists wishing to update their knowledge of oculoplastic surgery. It aims to provide a practical guide to the management of basic oculoplastic problems. It does not try to give didactic details of a systematic series of surgical procedures, but rather to present an outline of the different options which are available to the surgeon with their advantages and disadvantages. This is achieved by a team of contributors practising in different countries throughout the world who have all worked at Moorfields Eye Hospital with the editors, but who have adapted their practice to their current local circumstances. In this way we hope to have provided a surgical guide which will be of value throughout the world.

Richard Collin
Geoffrey Rose

1 Anatomy and general considerations

Fiona Robinson

A sound understanding of the basic anatomy of the eyelids, lacrimal system and orbits is essential in order to perform successful surgery. This chapter presents a basic overview together with general considerations relative to oculoplastic and orbital surgery.

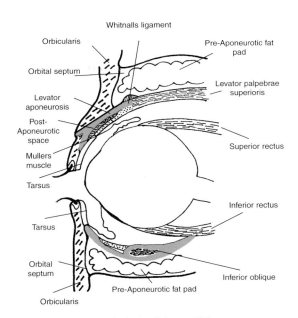

Figure 1.1   Sagittal view of the eyelid structures.

The eyelids

The eyelids may be divided into anterior and posterior lamellae. The anterior leaf is composed of skin and orbicularis and the posterior of tarsus and conjunctiva. The "grey line" of the lid margin marks the separation between conjunctiva which covers tarsus and squamous epithelium which covers orbicularis. In plastic surgery, procedures are often described as involving the anterior or posterior lamella.

The upper lid margin lies 1 to 2mm below the superior limbus, the peak lying just nasal to the centre of the pupil. The lower lid margin sits at the corneal limbus, its lowest portion lying slightly temporal to the pupil. The upper lid crease is 8 to 12mm above the lashes and is formed by the subcutaneous insertion of the terminal fibres of the levator aponeurosis. The lower lid crease is more poorly defined as there are no subcutaneous insertions corresponding to those of the upper eyelid. The nasojugal fold extends inferior and laterally from the medial canthal angle along the side of the nose and the angular blood vessels will generally be located in this fold.

Skin

Eyelid skin is thin allowing good mobility of the eyelids. In part due to this thinness, it has a tendency to stretch with age. The resultant excessive skin can be used for full thickness skin grafts. Such skin grafts take well as there is little subcutaneous fat. It should be noted that the lower lid has no vertical excess skin and one should excise lesions from the lower lid as vertically as possible to avoid a cicatricial ectropion.

1

Orbicularis

The orbicularis muscle surrounds the eye and closes the lids. The concentrically placed fibres are divided into three parts: the outer orbital and two inner palpebral portions – preseptal and pretarsal – and these contribute to the superficial and deep portions of the medial and lateral canthal tendons. Deep extensions at the medial canthus insert onto the fascia overlying the lacrimal sac and posterior lacrimal crest and aid in the lacrimal pump mechanism. When cut orbicularis fibres contract and pull skin edges apart. One must pull wound edges together before deciding on any lid repair.

Medical canthal tendon

This supports the nasal aspect of the eye lids. The anterior limb inserts onto the anterior lacrimal crest and beyond to the frontal process of the maxilla. The common canaliculus enters the lacrimal sac behind the anterior limb. The posterior limb inserts onto the posterior lacrimal crest and contributes most to the stability of the medial canthus. An attempt should always be made to reform this component in eyelid reconstruction. The vertical component is a fascial support that extends from the anterior limb to insert onto the frontal bone. One should check for medial canthal tendon laxity before deciding on management for any eyelid malposition.

Lateral canthal tendon

This supports and holds the lid posteriorly against the globe. It consists of a superior and inferior limb and is the tendon of origin of the pretarsal orbicularis. A ligamentous element is due to a direct extension from the tarsus. It inserts at Whitnall's tubercle, 2mm posterior to the lateral orbital rim. It is important to maintain at least one limb of the lateral canthal tendon in any eyelid reconstruction.

Orbital septum

The septum is a tough inelastic sheet of fibrous tissue that divides the eyelids from the orbit. It is a multilaminated structure that arises from the orbital rim (arcus marginalis) and attaches loosely to the eyelid retractors. It acts as an important barrier to the spread of infection from the lids to the orbit.

Pre-aponeurotic fat pad

Lying behind the orbital septum and in front of the retractors is the pre-aponeurotic fat pad. Knowledge of its position is invaluable in identifying the retractors during surgery. The upper lid has nasal and central fat pads and care must be taken to distinguish the latter from the lacrimal gland.

Upper lid retractors

These consist of three distinct parts forming one unit which lifts the eyelid. The levator palpebrae superioris is a striated muscle that arises from the lesser wing of the sphenoid directly above the Annulus of Zinn in the posterior orbit. It runs forward under the orbital roof for 40mm before changing direction and splitting into two elements, the anteriorly placed aponeurosis and a thin strip of smooth muscle (Müller's).

The aponeurosis is a dense sheet of collagen fibres that runs towards the lid margin and inserts onto the anterior surface of the tarsal plate and also between orbicularis fibres anteriorly to form the skin crease. The aponeurosis also fans out medially and laterally into the horns. The lateral horn splits the lacrimal gland into orbital and palpebral lobes and inserts onto Whitnall's tubercle. The medial horn attaches to the medial orbital wall. Müller's muscle extends from the levator below the aponeurosis and in front of conjunctiva down to the tarsus and attaches to the superior edge of the tarsus by a 1mm tendon.

Whitnall's ligament (superior transverse ligament)

Whitnall's ligament is a fascial condensation that stretches horizontally across the orbit between the trochlea medially, and lacrimal gland fascia laterally supporting the levator complex. It is at the level of Whitnall's that the levator begins to transform into its aponeurotic extension 10 to 12mm above the tarsus.

Lower lid retractors

Although the upper and lower lids are analogous structures the main distinction is the lid retractors. While the upper lid gains tremendous mobility through the striated levator muscle, the lower lid gains most of its movement via a fibrous extension from the inferior rectus muscle with a range of only 3 to 5mm. The lower lid retractors consist of a sheet of fibrous tissue which extends from the inferior rectus sheath, splits to encapsulate inferior oblique and then runs forward to the inferior tarsal border accompanied by some strips of smooth muscle (inferior tarsal muscle).

Tarsal plates

The superior and inferior tarsal plates provide stability to the upper and lower eyelids. Provided the tarsus is healthy, only 4mm height is needed for stability and therefore tarsal tissue from the upper eyelid (10mm) can be used as a graft to re-construct the lower eyelid (3–4mm) or the other upper eyelid. The meibomian glands are found within the tarsal plates.

The lacrimal system

Secretory system

The lacrimal gland is an exocrine gland and lies in the anterior superolateral quadrant of the orbit in the lacrimal fossa. It measures $20 \times 12 \times 5$mm and consists of orbital and palpebral lobes, the two being divided by the lateral horn of the levator aponeurosis. All of the ductules from the orbital lobe pass through the palpebral lobe and empty into the superior conjunctival fornix, 5mm above the superolateral border of the tarsus. The accessory lacrimal glands of Krause are located in the fornices and the glands of Wolfring are found at the upper and lower tarsal borders of the superior and inferior tarsus respectively.

Excretory system (Figure 1.2)

The puncta on the medial aspect of the upper and lower lid margins mark the opening of the lacrimal drainage system. Each leads into a 2mm vertical dilatation of the canaliculus (ampulla) followed by an 8 to 10mm horizontal portion. It is important to recognise this canalicular configuration when performing tear sac wash-out and to hold the lid taut during the procedure. The superior and inferior canaliculus combine to form the common canaliculus which leads into the lacrimal sac. Its entry into the sac is normally partially covered by a flap of mucosa (Valve of Rosenmüller).

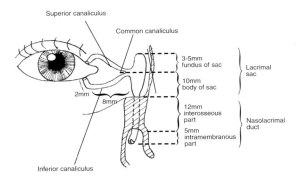

Figure 1.2   Lacrimal drainage system.

The lacrimal sac leads into the nasolacrimal duct. The duct has an upper intraosseous (12mm) segment, the direction of which is inferior and slightly lateral and posterior. The lower intramembranous segment (5mm) opens into the lateral wall of the nose beneath the inferior turbinate. The ostium is covered by a mucosal valve (of Hasner). The tear flow is actively pumped from the tear lake by the actions of the orbicularis muscle (Figure 1.3).

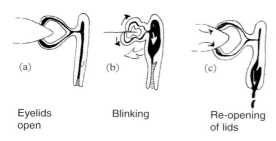

| (a) | (b) | (c) |
| Eyelids open | Blinking | Re-opening of lids |

Figure 1.3 The lacrimal pump.

The orbit

The bony orbit (Figure 1.4)

The orbit lies behind the orbital septum. It has four walls composed of seven bones; ethmoid, frontal, lacrimal, maxillary, palatine, sphenoid and zygomatic. The walls (roof, lateral, medial, floor) taper posteriorly to the apex and optic canal. The medial orbital walls are approximately 1cm apart and parallel, and the adult orbit volume is 30cc. Each orbit wall has particular important relations. The roof has the anterior cranial fossa and frontal sinus above. The medial wall has adjacent nasal cavity, ethmoid sinuses and more posterior sphenoid sinus. The maxillary antrum is beneath the floor. The lateral wall is located adjacent to the middle cranial fossa, temporal fossa and pterygopalatine fossa. The thinnest bone is in the medial wall (lamina papyracea) adjacent to the ethmoid air cells. The floor is also thin especially medially and these are the areas most frequently fragmented in "blow out" fractures. The orbital walls are perforated by several significant apertures. The Annulus of Zinn is a fibrous ring formed by the common origin of the four rectus muscles. The relationships of the superior orbital fissure, inferior orbital fissure, Annulus of Zinn and optic foramen and their contents are shown in Figure 1.5.

Surgical spaces

The orbit may be divided into three surgical "spaces". The potential subperiosteal space lies between the bone and the periorbita. The intra and extraconal spaces are divided by the extraocular muscles and intermuscular septa.

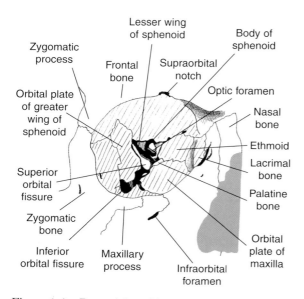

Figure 1.4 Bony right orbit.

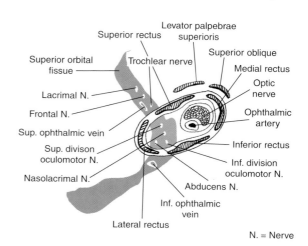

Figure 1.5 Annulus of Zinn and related structures.

The subperiosteal space provides an easily dissectable plane for surgical access and follows the contours of the orbital walls. The most important structure in the extraconal space is the lacrimal gland. Within the muscle cone, i.e. in the intraconal space, lies orbital fat, the optic nerve plus blood vessels and nerves.

Blood supply, nerve supply and lymphatic drainage

The internal and external carotid arteries supply blood to the eyelids and orbit with rich anastomoses between the two. This good blood supply accounts for rapid healing and relative lack of infection. The venous drainage generally follows the arterial supply. There are no identifiable lymphatic vessels in the orbit. Medial lymphatics of the eyelids drain to the submandibular lymph nodes, the lateral group to the preauricular nodes. The sensory innervation of the eyelids and orbit is via the ophthalmic and maxillary divisions of the Trigeminal nerve.

General considerations for surgery

Patient preparation and intraoperative care

Proper patient selection, adequate pre-operative assessment and meticulous surgical techniques optimise surgical outcome. The patient should be properly informed as to the type of procedure, benefit of procedure and potential complications. As far as possible the surgeon should decide pre-operatively the procedure of choice and obtain patient consent prior to the day of surgery.

Intraoperatively, trauma to tissues is minimised by the use of specialised instruments (for example skin hooks) and careful handling of soft tissue. Appropriate sutures and needle points lead to best wound closure and healing.

Anaesthesia

Anaesthetic options available to the patient are local, local with sedation and general. The choice is individual to each patient. Local infiltration allows for patient co-operation, rapid recovery time and accuracy in lid surgery. It is reliable and rarely needs the addition of a regional block although the latter is necessary in lacrimal drainage surgery. The anaesthetic agent may be short or long acting or a combination of both. The addition of adrenaline gives vasoconstriction, prolonged anaesthesia and better haemostasis if given 10 minutes to act. The injection is subcutaneous avoiding visible vessels and penetration of muscle to minimise haematoma formation.

Indications for general anaesthetic are diminishing. It is usually reserved for more invasive orbital procedures and eyelid surgery on children.

Incisions

All skin incisions result in scar formation. Scars are less obvious if the incision is made in or parallel to skin creases, for example an upper eye lid incision in the upper lid crease for ptosis surgery

If this is not possible one should try to keep the incision parallel to the lines of minimum skin tension (Figure 1.6). One exception to this is the vertical incision for lower lid lesions to avoid cicatricial ectropion. The incision should be as vertical as possible for the smallest scar and rapid healing. It is always helpful to mark an incision before distortion by local anaesthetic or stretching and it should be made in a single steady motion. It is helpful to cut "down-hill to uphill" to avoid blood obscuring the surgical field.

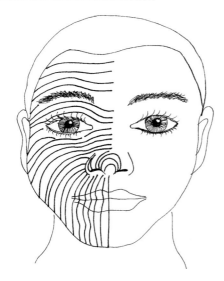

Figure 1.6   Lines of minimum skin tension.

Further reading

Collin JRO. *A Manual of Systematic Eyelid Surgery* (2nd ed). London: Churchill Livingstone, 1989.

Jones LT, Wobig JL. *Surgery of the Eyelids and Lacrimal System*. Aesculapius, 1976.

McCord CD, Tanenbaum M, Nunery WR. *Oculoplastic Surgery* (3rd ed). New York: Raven Press, 1995.

McNab AA. *Manual of Orbital and Lacrimal Surgery*. Edinburgh: Churchill Livingstone, 1994.

Zide BM, Jelks EW. *Surgery Anatomy of The Orbit*. New York: Raven Press, 1985.

2 Eyelid trauma and basic principles of reconstruction

John Pitts

A doctor's first introduction to ocular plastic surgery is often being called upon to repair an acute eyelid laceration. The management of both acute and chronic or established eyelid injuries is laid out in this chapter. Surgical repair depends on a knowledge of eyelid anatomy and of the principles of eyelid reconstruction which are described here.

The advanced trauma life support system (ALTS) was developed by the American College of Surgeons in 1993 as an algorithmic approach to the management of patients with life-threatening injuries. It is important that everyone involved in the early resuscitation of the injured patient has the same priorities regardless of specialty.

ATLS can be stated simply as:

- rapid primary survey
- simultaneous resuscitation
- detailed secondary survey
- appropriate referral
- patient transfer
- definitive care.

The involvement of the oculoplastic surgeon is likely to begin when the patient has been stabilised and the detailed secondary survey has revealed orbital trauma. Other specialties may be involved in patients with craniofacial trauma and it is important that the priorities for repair are decided and a treatment plan adopted early. For example, it is important to repair a ruptured globe before major bone manipulations are carried out in the definitive repair of facial fractures, but it would be unreasonable to delay the treatment of torrential haemorrhage or severe neurosurgical injury in the same circumstances.

Principles of soft tissue repair

Antitetanus prophylaxis

Details are given in Table 2.1

Table 2.1 Guidelines for antitetanus prophylaxis.

Immunisation status	Clean wounds	Tetanus-prone wounds
Last injection of a course or booster within 10 years	Nil	Nil or booster if high risk of infection
Last injection of a course or booster more than 10 years previously	Antitetanus toxoid	Antitetanus toxoid and human antitetanus immunoglobulin (inject at different sites)
Not immunised or status unknown	Primary course of antitetanus toxoid	Primary course of antitetanus toxoid and human antitetanus immunoglobulin (inject at different sites)

Removal of dirt and foreign bodies

This is carried out to reduce the risk of infection and prevent tattooing of the tissues. The cornea is protected using a lid guard and the tissues scrubbed using a sterile hand scrub brush. Larger fragments are removed individually with forceps. The area is irrigated with saline and the process repeated until all visible contaminants are removed. Adequate retraction of wounds is important, and the operating microscope is helpful in detecting smaller particulate contamination.

Preservation of tissues

Minimal surgical debridement is the rule in facial and lid lacerations due to the superior healing characteristics of wounds in this area, arising from its abundant blood supply.

Principles of wound closure

These are as follows:

- Use a simple everting technique (Figure 2.1).
- Approximate, don't strangulate.
- Use mattress sutures, over bolsters if necessary, where tissues are under tension and this cannot be fully relieved.
- Sutures should be placed at 2/3mm intervals and should be of uniform depth.

- Start to remove sutures early (3–5 days). Alternate suture removal is a useful technique to avoid scarring. Support the tissues with Steristrips over tincture of benzoin to promote adhesion.
- Avoid complex procedures in primary repair.

Sutures and needles

The main sutures used in oculoplastic repair are:

nylon 6/0

- non absorbable polyamide synthetic fibre
- 10mm reverse cutting needle

5/0 and 6/0 silk

- non absorbable protein fibre
- 10mm reverse cutting needle

5/0 and 6/0 Vicryl or Dexon

- polyglactin 910 braided monofilament
- absorbed in 70 days
- provides wound support for 30 days
- 8mm half-circle spatulated needle

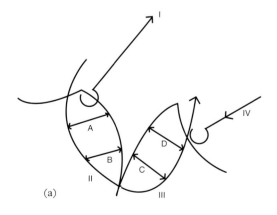 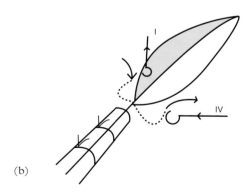

Figure 2.1   Technique for producing an everted skin wound.
(a) The skin hook (I) pulls the entry site skin edge upwards. The needle trajectory (II) takes a greater bite of tissue in the midsection of the wound (B) than in the superficial section (A) of the flap. The curve of the skin hook (IV) then presses on the exit site skin edge. The needle trajectory (III) takes a greater bite of tissue in the midsection of the wound (C) than in the superficial section (D) of the flap.
(b) This shows the desired roll of tissue produced. Remember: on entry, pull skin edge upwards. On exit, push tissue downwards.

Box 2.1 Instruments for oculoplastic repair

A basic set for oculoplastic repair should include:
- Suction and bipolar cautery systems
- Clarkes, guarded or Barraquers lid speculum
- Stallard (shoe horn) lid guard
- Desmarres retractors
- Rollets catspaw retractors
- Gillies skin hooks
- Squint hooks
- Caliper, rule and marker pen

Needle holders:
- Silcocks self-retaining
- Troutman or Barraquers non-locking

Toothed forceps:
- St Martins
- Jayles
- Listers
- Adsons

Non-toothed forceps:
- Moorfields

Haemostats:
- Spencer-Wells artery forceps
- Mosquito forceps

Straight scissors:
- Sharp-ended
- Blunt-ended

Curved Scissors:
- Enucleation
- Westcott spring scissors

Lacrimal:
- Hayes seeker/Nettleships dilator
- Bowmans probes

Note: 6/0 Vicryl rapide, which is absorbed in 42 days and which provides wound support for 10 days, is useful for skin closure in children. Vicryl used for skin closure should be undyed to avoid tattooing.

5/0 ethibond

- braided polybutylate coated polyester
- non-absorbable; remains encapsulated in tissue
- 8mm half-circle spatulated needle.

Types of specific wounds

Bite wounds

Bite wounds are always contaminated and are often associated with tissue loss. Direct closure should be attempted after thorough cleaning and tetanus prophylaxis, metronidazole, and a broad spectrum antibiotic to cover eikenella for human bites and pasturella for animal bites.

Stab wounds

The dimensions of the weapon should be used to give an idea of whether frontocranial perforation is likely and CT scans used whenever this possibility is considered. The wound should be explored to identify damaged structures. Superficial wounds should be cleaned and primary closure obtained. Antitetanus prophylaxis should be given according to the protocol.

If a weapon remains in position it should not be removed until there are full resuscitative and operative facilities available including cross-matched blood and neurosurgical expertise. Plain films in two orthogonal planes and CT scanning are useful in demonstrating the position of the weapon, but angiography may be necessary where damage to major vessels is suspected.

When the instrument is removed there is a period of initial brisk haemorrhage which then subsides. Vascular clips, ties and cautery help to control haemorrhage, and Surgicel can be packed along the track of the wound. There is a risk of secondary haemorrhage when the blood volume is restored and the patient begins to mobilise.

Eyelid lacerations

Delay in repair is acceptable while more life-threatening injuries are dealt with, but it is important to ensure that the globe is protected from pressure until penetrating injury is excluded, and the cornea is protected from dehydration until the lids can be repaired. One should always check for penetrating injury when the patient is under general anaesthetic before embarking on repair of eyelid lacerations.

If the globe is intact, or when it has been repaired, lid lacerations should be repaired. This should be performed before repair of other facial lacerations, because primary closure in circumstances where tissue loss has occurred elsewhere in the face may result in stretching and difficult closure in the periocular region. The upper lid takes priority and should be repaired before the lower lid. Avoid excising tissue from the eyelids, as even apparently devitalised tissues may regain perfusion when anatomical relationships have been restored. In repairing the lids, it is important that the tarsal plates are accurately aligned to prevent eyelid deformity, and the eyelid margins must be smooth to prevent corneal damage.

Closure of eyelid lacerations

The method of closure is detailed here.

- Place a lid guard to protect the globe.
- Align the grey line with 6/0 virgin silk. Leave the ends long and place the suture under light traction to bring the tarsal plates into alignment.

- Close the tarsal plate with 5/0 Vicryl. These are structural sutures and the bites must be tested for adequacy and placed just shallow to the conjunctival plane to avoid rubbing on the cornea.
- Close skin and orbicularis with 6/0 silk or nylon.
- Release the grey line suture from traction and tie it down away from the cornea with the top skin suture.
- Remove skin sutures at day five.
- Remove the grey line suture at day ten.

Lacerations parallel to the orbicularis fibres

These do not gape and can be left if small. Larger, slightly gaping wounds can be closed with a subcuticular technique.

Lacerations perpendicular to the orbicularis fibres

These have a tendency to gape and healing by primary intention leaves an unsightly scar, producing distortion of the eyelid margin and poor functional results. The obicularis should be closed with interrupted 6/0 catgut sutures. The skin is closed with 6/0 silk or nylon using an everting technique.

Lacerations to the levator muscle

The levator can consistently be found under the pre-aponeurotic fat pad and the severed ends brought into apposition using 6/0 catgut or Vicryl. Lacerations of the levator aponeurosis will heal spontaneously if less than half of its width is involved.

When the levator muscle is severely damaged it may be easier to perform an accurate primary repair of other lid structures and repair the levator as a secondary procedure under local anaesthesia, using the movement of the muscle in upgaze to help identify the proximal end.

Prevention of amblyopia

In orbital trauma in children it is important to take steps to prevent amblyopia by measures aimed at reducing swelling rapidly (ice packs, prompt treatment of infection) and occluding the fellow eye if necessary. While it would be acceptable to delay the repair of a traumatic ptosis in an adult, this would carry the risk of amblyopia in a child and a temporary brow suspension should be carried out urgently if necessary. It is preferable to use a non-integratible material for the suspension such as a prolene suture or silicone rod so that it can be removed subsequently if the ptosis recovers.

Tissue loss

It is preferable to avoid adding tissue in a primary repair unless the globe would otherwise be exposed. In any eyelid reconstruction the lid should be considered as consisting of an anterior lamella of skin and orbicularis muscle and a posterior lamella of tarsus and conjunctiva. Both lamellae can be reformed either with a flap or a graft. A flap is preferable as it usually provides better cosmesis, but especially after trauma a suitable flap may not be easily available. Full-thickness skin grafts are preferable to split-thickness skin unless the defect is very large, there is insufficient full-thickness skin available or the bed of the graft is poor, for example after burns. Skin grafts added at the time of the primary repair after trauma tend to scar more than if they are used to correct a cicatricial ectropion and scar as a secondary procedure (*vide infra*).

Posterior lamella defects can be corrected with a flap of conjunctiva or tarsoconjunctiva or with a graft of tarsus, conjunctiva, mucosa from the lip/cheek, hard palate or nasal septum with its attached mucoperichondrium. As with anterior lamella reconstruction it is preferable to delay posterior lamella reconstruction after trauma and treat any entropion (Chapter 4) as a secondary procedure unless corneal exposure cannot be controlled. The same principles govern the timing of full-thickness eyelid reconstruction (Chapter 6). The procedure of choice after trauma depends on the remaining viable tissue and with a second stage procedure, on the position of the scars.

Medial canthal lacerations

These are commonly seen in dog bites. The medial canthus may be avulsed and canalicular lacerations often coexist.

Anterior limb

If only the anterior limb is damaged, then this can be approximated using 6/0 ethibond.

Posterior limb

If the posterior limb is involved in the injury then repair of the anterior limb alone will result in eversion of the medial end of the eyelid. The medial end of the tarsal plate should be sutured to the periosteum of the posterior lacrimal crest provided that an adequate fixation point is present. If no adequate fixation point can be found then a miniplate or transnasal wiring technique can be used.

Canalicular lacerations

In discussing the controversy which surrounds the management of canalicular lacerations, it is important to remember that under normal circumstances, 30% of the tear drainage is via the upper and 70% via the lower canaliculus. Some authors, particularly in the USA, consider that all lacerations of the canaliculi should be repaired using the technique of intubation of the whole nasolacrimal apparatus. Other authorities point out that epiphora is rare unless both canaliculi are involved, and that isolated injury of either the upper or the lower canaliculus is likely to be compensated for by the other canaliculus. It follows that no method of repair which compromises the function of the undamaged canaliculus should be contemplated. If the decision is made to repair a single canalicular injury, then this should be carried out using the operating microscope. 8/0 Vicryl sutures are used to approximate the ends of the canaliculus over a 1mm silicone stent, which is sutured to the lid margin and removed after two weeks. The canaliculus must be regularly dilated to keep it open. Although this method has the advantage of not involving the uninjured canaliculus, Welham points out that it is unlikely to remain patent and carries the risk of producing lid distortion and ectropion. In the light of these considerations, the following recommendations are made.

- *Bicanalicular lacerations* should be repaired using an intubation technique but the patient must be warned that post operative stenosis is likely and that this may subsequently require conjunctivo-dacryocystorhinostomy (DCR) with placement of a Pyrex tube.
- *Single canalicular lacerations* can be dealt with safely by accurately repairing the eyelid, ensuring apposition to the globe, and marsupialising the distal segment of the transected canaliculus in the wound using a three-snip procedure. The marsupialised area can be held open by placing 8/0 Vicryl sutures.
- *Common canalicular lacerations* are dealt with by carrying out a primary canaliculo-DCR with intubation.
- *Lacrimal sac lacerations* are treated by a DCR (Dacryocystorhinostomy) with intubation as a primary procedure.

Indications for primary removal of globe

Primary enucleation to prevent the development of sympathetic ophthalmia is no longer advocated. Where possible, the injured eye should undergo accurate primary repair until the intraocular damage can be assessed in detail. Modern intraocular surgery can often salvage severely damaged eyes. If there is no visual potential after an ocular perforating injury, the ocular inflammatory reaction does not settle down rapidly or the eye has been grossly disrupted, it is wise to carry out an enucleation as a secondary procedure, preferably within two to four weeks of the trauma.

Management of scarring

Healing wounds in the acute phase should be held in apposition with sutures to minimise the blood clot and fibrin. After two weeks fibroblast activity increases and the wound enters the contraction phase which lasts about twelve weeks. It can be influenced by various factors including pressure, massage, steroids, anti-mitotic agents such as Mitomycin C, and vitamins such as Vitamin E and C. After twelve weeks the scar enters the phase of maturation and the fibroblasts become aligned. Activity can be monitored by the redness and thickness in the scar. If a wound is unsatisfactory it can be opened and re-sutured in the first two weeks. After that the fibroblast activity is intense and any scar revision is likely to be complicated by an excessive response. The scars should be left until they are judged to be "mature" which means they are no longer thick or red. This will certainly take three months, even after a clean primary surgical would, and after trauma it may take six to nine months or longer.

The principles of scar revision of a mature scar are to excise the scar itself, preferably to break up the line of the scar e.g. with a Z-plasty or (Figure 2.2) multiple Z-plasties, and to re-suture it as accurately as possible with relief of all tension. Pressure, massage, steroids, etc. can be used post operatively to modify the scar healing as desired.

Cicatricial ectropion

This is diagnosed by pushing the lower eyelid upwards. Normally it will reach the margin of the upper lid with the eye open. Less severe degrees can be demonstrated by asking the patient to open his/her mouth. The tension in the lower eyelid skin will pull the lid margin away from the globe.

The treatment of cicatricial ectropion depends on whether it is due to a vertical linear scar or to a combined more generalised horizontal and vertical skin shortage.

Z-Plasty (Figure 2.2)

Z-plasty is used as follows to treat vertical scars.

- The lid is placed on traction using a mattress stitch over tarsorrhaphy tubing.
- The scar is marked along its length.
- The upper and lower limbs of the Z are marked.
- A single Z can be converted to multiple Zs.
- The skin flaps are raised and reflected on skin hooks.
- Underlying cicatrix is excised and haemostasis obtained.
- The flaps are transposed and sutured in place "A-stitches" are useful at the apices of the flaps (Figure 2.3).
- The lid is placed on traction.
- Pressure dressings are applied for 48 hours.

Skin grafting

This is used to treat combined horizontal and vertical skin shortage.

- The lid is placed on upward traction.
- A subciliary incision is made and the skin reflected from the underlying orbicularis until the lower lid margin can lie in contact with the upper lid margin in its open position. This will produce an oversized graft bed to compensate for subsequent contraction.

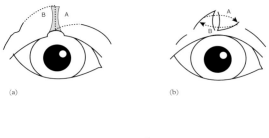

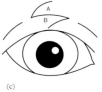

Figure 2.2   Z-plasty. The central limb of the Z is placed along the line of the scar. The limbs are equal in length. The optimal angle between the limbs is 60°. Z-plasty produces a gain in length along the common limb of the original Z. For 60° angles the gain is 75%. It also produces a 90° change in the orientation of the common limb of the Z. In the example shown, the Z can be designed to hide a scar in the upper lid skin crease.

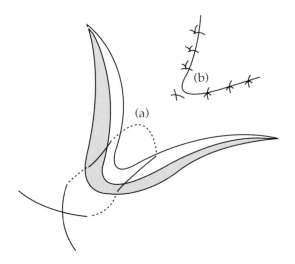

Figure 2.3   The A-suture for placing the apex of a V-shaped wound. (a) shows the subcutaneous path of the suture through the apex of the triangular flap. (b) shows the tied suture approximating the apex of the flap in the V of the wound and subsequent everting sutures.

- The graft bed is blotted with paper conveniently obtained from the suture pack.

- The paper is trimmed around the blotted area to produce a template of the graft required.
- The template is placed on the donor site and a marker pen used to draw its outline.
- Suitable donor sites include the pre-auricular skin, the post-auricular skin and the supraclavicular fossa.
- The donor site is infiltrated with xylocaine/adrenaline.
- The donor skin is raised using skin hooks and a number 15 Bard Parker blade and wrapped in sterile saline soaked gauze.
- The edges of the donor site may be undermined to allow closure without undue tension.
- The donor skin is everted over the surgeon's finger and subcutaneous fat trimmed off. Trimming must not be excessive, to avoid damage to the vascular plexus.
- Small horizontal incisions can be made to allow tissue fluid egress if desired.
- The graft is trimmed and sutured in place with anchoring sutures; these can be left long-ended to support external bolsters if desired.
- The definitive graft sutures are placed; a continuous Vicryl rapide or tissue glue can be used in situations where subsequent suture removal may be problematic (in children, for example).
- Additional support can be achieved by passing double-armed sutures through the lid and graft and tying these through tarsorrhaphy tubing.
- The lid is placed on upward traction.
- External bolsters are fashioned from gauze to match the graft and tied in place with the long-ended anchoring sutures.
- Pressure dressings are applied and left in place for 48 hours.

Dermis-fat grafting

Dermis-fat grafts are useful in supplying subcutaneous bulk to scarred areas in the lower lid/cheek and in the upper lid sulcus. The fat cells inhibit further scarring and provide a more natural antifibrotic effect than antimetabolites.

Dermis-fat grafts can be obtained from the periumbilical and groin regions of the abdomen or from the buttock. The graft is marked and xylocaine/adrenaline injected to obtain a *peau d'orange* effect. The epidermis is raised and excised using a blade in a manner similar to raising a split-skin graft, then discarded. The dermis-fat graft is excised and placed in sterile, saline-soaked gauze while the donor site is closed. The dermal element can be sutured into the scarred tissues such that it supports the fat element which comes to lie subcutaneously.

Further reading

Canavan M, Archer DB. Long term review of injuries to the lacrimal apparatus. *Trans Ophthalmol Soc UK* 1979; **63**:549–55.

Collin JRO. Repair of eyelid injuries. In: *Manual of systematic eyelid surgery*. Edinburgh: Churchill Livingstone, 1989.

Dryden RN, Beyer TL. Repair of canalicular lacerations with silicone intubation. In: Levine MR. *Manual of oculoplastic surgery*. New York: Churchill Livingstone, 1988.

Mansour MA, Moore EE, Moore FA, Whitehill TA. Validating the selective management of penetrating neck wounds. *Am J Surg* 1991; **162**:517–21.

Mustarde J. *Repair and reconstruction in the orbital region: a practical guide*. Edinburgh: Churchill Livingstone, 1980.

Saunders DH. The effectiveness of the pigtail probe method of repairing canalicular lacerations. *Ophthalmic Surg* 1978; **9**:33–9.

Welham RAN. The lacrimal apparatus. In: Miller S. *Clinical ophthalmology*. London: Wright, 1987.

3 Ectropion

Michèle Beaconsfield

The term ectropion is derived from the Greek *ek* (away from) and *tropein* (to turn) and refers to any form of everted lid margin.

The eyelid margin position is dependent on the tension in the tarsus and the canthal tendons (Figure 3.1), supported by the orbicularis muscle. Spasm of the orbicularis, as may occur in new born infants, can cause spontaneous eversion of the lids. Ageing changes affecting the orbicularis muscle and the canthal tendons are the cause of involutional ectropion. This is aggravated by the laxity of the lower lid retractors. Tumours, such as meibomian cysts, may cause mechanical ectropion. Cicatricial ectropion is caused by a shortage of skin. This may be congenital, as in some patients with Down's syndrome, or acquired following trauma; it may involve the upper and/or the lower lid. In seventh nerve palsy and paralytic ectropion, the support normally provided by the orbicularis muscle is absent: the lower lid position is therefore dependent on the medial and lateral canthal tendons which stretch mechanically with time.

Although classifications are helpful, many ectropia are multifactorial. Thus what started as a cicatricial ectropion, with shortage of skin, may progress to include stretching of the tarsus and canthal tendons. Only correcting the skin shortage may in itself be insufficient: a lid tightening procedure may be required, in addition to addressing the skin shortage, to adequately correct the ectropion. The most important factors to establish in corrective surgery are where and how the lid should be tightened or supported. This forms the basis of this chapter. The correction of other factors involved in ectropion repair is covered elsewhere, such as skin shortage (Chapter 2) and seventh nerve palsy (Chapter 7).

Ectropion is classified as:

- Congenital
- Acquired
  - Involutional
  - Mechanical
  - Cicatricial
  - Paralytic

Congenital ectropion

This may be acute, as a result of spasm of the orbicularis muscle as seen in the new-born infant, or established by skin shortage such as may occur in some cases of children with Down's syndrome. Orbicularis spasm is managed by gently repositioning the everted lids with a finger and lubricating the exposed conjunctiva with antibiotic ointment. Rarely, inverting sutures are required (*vide infra*).

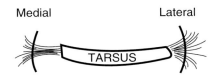

Medial   Lateral

TARSUS

Figure 3.1   Lower lid margin elements. Tarsus and canthal tendons.

Established congenital ectropion due to skin shortage may result in corneal exposure problems. These can usually be managed with lubricants but if this proves insufficient then skin grafting may be undertaken (Chapter 2). Lid tightening procedures may also be required (*vide infra*).

Acquired ectropion

Looking at the patient can often reveal signs which will help to define the ectropion such as a mass pulling the lid down, or hemifacial sagging with the inability to close the eye as seen in seventh nerve palsy. In involutional medial ectropion, the lower punctum may be seen to evert and override the upper lid margin only on blinking.

Palpation further indicates aetiology. Pushing the cheek skin up to the lower orbital rim with a finger relieves skin shortage, thus confirming the suspicion of cicatricial ectropion. In the absence of skin shortage and tumours, and with normal lid closure, the ectropion is likely to be due to lid laxity. The next point to establish is where the lid is maximally lax (medially/centrally/laterally) and this is judged by gently pulling on the lid in the various directions to determine the possible amount and direction of displacement. It is worth noting if there is excess skin: this can be excised at the time of surgery. Finally, if the conjunctiva has been exposed for any length of time it may be inflamed or even chemotic. There may be crusting due to drying of secretions and even keratinisation. It may be necessary to insert temporary inverting sutures to pull the conjunctiva back down and into the fornix to restore its normal anatomical position: this will contribute greatly to improving its surface and to reducing oedema.

Involutional ectropion

It is now understood that various factors contribute to the generalised sagging of the lower lid including medial canthal tendon laxity, tarsal sagging, lateral canthal tendon laxity, and the less common laxity/loss of attachment of the lower lid retractors to the lower border of the tarsus. Initially the latter results in loss of the lower lid skin crease on downgaze and ultimately leads to total tarsal eversion. What determines whether the lax lid turns in or out is the movement of the preseptal band of orbicularis muscle. This is still well tethered in ectropion and does not roll upwards over the lower border of the tarsus, as in involutional entropion (Chapter 4).

Central ectropion

Patients are often diagnosed with conjunctivitis/discharge and treated with topical antibiotics. The symptoms recur the moment these are stopped. This is probably because the dryness of the exposed conjunctiva is temporarily alleviated with the lubrication of the antibiotics, thereby stemming the apparent "discharge" produced to protect the exposure. While waiting for surgery, it is not unreasonable to sparingly lubricate the exposed tarsal conjunctiva with two to three times daily application of simple eye ointment or equivalent. This will keep the surface moist without contaminating the corneal surface and fogging the vision.

Central ectropion describes a sag downwards and/or outwards of the lid margin, without associated canthal tendon laxity. When the lid is pulled away and forward from the globe it does not spring or snap back to the globe as crisply as a taut tarsus. This laxity is traditionally corrected with a full thickness pentagon excision. Bick originally described a pentagon excision at the lateral extremity of the tarsus with reattachment to the lateral canthus. The modified Bick procedure of *full thickness pentagon excision and direct closure*, just under a quarter of the way in from the lateral canthus, is now the standard correction for central ectropion. It is very successful in the absence of medial or lateral canthal laxity.

The vertical incision through the tarsus should be made about 5 mm from the lateral canthal corner, so that the reconstruction does not, even after resection, rub on the corner. The amount of lid to be resected is determined by overlapping the cut edges until the margin is taut. The tissue inferior to the tarsus is excised as a triangle, thus completing the pentagon (Figure 3.2a). The meticulous apposition of the tarsal edges, with long acting absorbable sutures, dictates the appearance and strength of the final result (Figure 3.2b). Accurate marginal closure is secured with grey line and lash line sutures; after tying, the trailing ends are kept long and secured in the tying of the first skin suture before trimming. This avoids any cut ends, which may be too short, rubbing on the eye (Figure 3.2c).

If there is considerable excess skin, the above procedure can be combined with a lower lid blepharoplasty (*Kuhnt-Symanovsky type procedure*): excess skin is excised as a

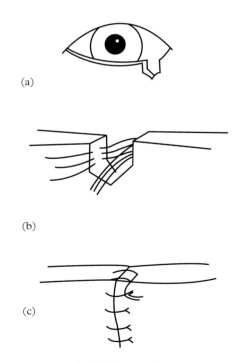

(a)

(b)

(c)

Figure 3.2   Modified Bick procedure.
(a) Pentagon excision, (b) Tarsal closure, (c) margin and skin closure.

lateral triangle from a blepharoplasty flap and the pentagon excision to shorten the horizontal laxity is done under the flap.

Lateral ectropion

These patients often complain of tear overflow laterally. When the lid margin is pulled forwards and medially, the lateral canthal corner seems to follow the pull and can be dragged to the extent that the laxity of the lower limb of the lateral canthal tendon will allow. In an intact lateral canthal tendon, there is an immediate resistant tug that appears to refuse to let go of the orbital wall. Lateral canthal laxity is often associated with tarsal sag and poor snap-back response: these can be corrected with a *lateral tarsal strip*.

This procedure as described by Anderson is itself a modification of Tenzel's lateral canthal sling. The lateral canthal corner is opened with a horizontal incision, and the inferior limb of the lateral canthal tendon is exposed and divided. The medial end of the wound is lifted upwards and laterally to overlap the surgical site and determine how much horizontal shortening is required: this is where the new medial wound edge and strip will be. The strip is fashioned by clearing it of skin and orbicularis anteriorly, lash margin superiorly, and conjunctiva posteriorly. Conjunctiva is usually quite adherent to the tarsus and may need to be scraped off gently with something like a D15 blade. The inevitable venous ooze from this posterior surface is best controlled by pinching the tarsal strip in a damp gauze between finger and thumb for two minutes rather than jeopardise the integrity of the strip with aggressive cautery.

The newly fashioned strip is attached with a non-absorbable suture to the periosteum just inside the lateral orbital rim at the mid pupillary level (Figure 3.3), which places it just under the upper limb of the lateral canthal tendon. The mobilised anterior lamella is lifted up and out, as for a blepharoplasty, and

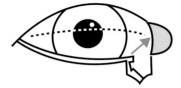

Figure 3.3   Lateral tarsal strip.

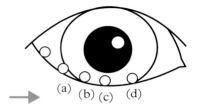

Figure 3.4   Lateral extent of punctal position in medial canthal laxity.

the estimated excess resected. Two or three long-acting, absorbable sutures secure the cut orbicularis: the long non-absorbable suture is thereby buried and the skin edges nearly apposed. Skin closure is standard.

Medial ectropion

Loss of lid margin apposition to the globe and resulting weakness of the physiological pump of blinking can lead to tear overflow. The repeated need to wipe aggravates the lid laxity. All patients with ectropion can present with epiphora, but this is more usual in those with mainly medial ectropion. The nasolacrimal outflow system should be syringed to elucidate any obstruction, as surgical correction of the ectropion alone will clearly not rid the patient of the symptoms in the presence of an obstruction; it will need to be combined with whatever lacrimal surgery is appropriate. Stenosis of the punctum only is common and secondary to drying and keratinisation. This usually resolves spontaneously over several weeks with reapposition to the globe.

Punctal eversion can be difficult to assess if mild, but is obvious on blinking. This may be observed as a single entity and repaired with a tarso-conjunctival diamond excision, or it may be associated with tarso-ligamentous laxity. The degree of medial canthal tendon laxity is estimated by gently pulling the lid laterally and watching how far the punctum can be dragged (Figure 3.4): not quite up to the medial limbus of the cornea is best repaired with a Lazy-T procedure (Figure 3.4a); past the limbus but not up to the pupil, indicating laxity of the anterior limb of the medial

canthal tendon, can be corrected with a plication (Figure 3.4b); to the mid pupillary line and needing posterior limb plication (Figure 3.4c); or past the pupil and beyond with obvious rounding of the previously pointed corner of the medial canthus: this indicates loss of the posterior limb of the medial canthal tendon which needs reattachment to the posterior lacrimal crest area (Figure 3.4d).

Punctal ectropion without horizontal laxity can be corrected by a modified Lester Jones *tarso-conjunctival diamond excision*, taken from the internal, i.e. conjunctival surface of the eyelid. The lid is everted for surgery by gently pulling on the 00 lacrimal probe that has been placed in the lower canaliculus. The tarsal component is present in the lateral half of the diamond (Figure 3.5a). A long-acting, absorbable suture is used to close the wound by apposing the north and south corners of the diamond. Before burying the knot, the lower lid retractors should be included in the suture (Figure 3.5b). This will prevent the punctum from pouting outwards on downgaze. The retractors are found by going into the diamond with a fine pair of toothed forceps and grabbing the surface lying anterior to the conjunctiva inferior to the lower border of the tarsus. The correct layer has been picked up if, on asking the patient to look down without moving the head, a tug is felt through the forceps.

If punctual ectropion is accompanied by tarsal laxity but the medial canthus is essentially intact, which is often the case, a

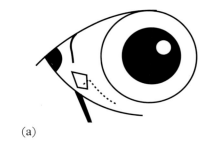

(a)

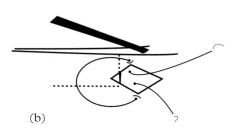

(b)

Figure 3.5 Modified Lester Jones tarso-conjunctival diamond excision. (a) tarso-conjunctival diamond excised; (b) tarsal surface view of closure (00 probe in canaliculus).

horizontal shortening procedure (full thickness pentagon excision) lateral to the punctum is combined with the tarsoconjunctival diamond excision, as in Smith's *Lazy T procedure*. The incision lines he described (horizontal below the punctum, and vertical through the lid) look like the letter T lying down resting, hence the suggestion that the T is being lazy (Figure 3.6).

If the laxity is medial to the punctum, i.e. within the medial canthal tendon, and the punctum can be pulled to the medial limbus of the cornea but not much beyond, the anterior limb of this tendon needs to be shortened. This can be achieved with a *plication of the anterior limb of the medial canthal tendon*. A horizontal skin incision is placed just below the lower canaliculus, which is held taut against the globe with a 00 lacrimal probe. The incision extends from just lateral to the punctum (to permit exposure of the medial edge of the tarsal plate) to just medial to the medial canthal corner. Through this incision the anterior limb of the medial canthal tendon is identified and exposed. A non-absorbable suture is passed

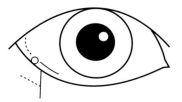

Figure 3.6 Lazy T.

through the medial end of the tarsus just below the level of the punctum and through the medial canthal tendon in a position that is superior and posterior to that of the tarsal stitch (Figure 3.7). The suture is tied tight enough to overcome the medial laxity, but not so much as to cause punctal eversion. The postero-superior positioning of the medial end of the stitch is important to avoid anterior displacement of the whole medial canthal corner, which would aggravate the ectropion rather than cure it.

If it is possible to pull the punctum laterally up to the pupil, it is the posterior limb of the medial canthal tendon that is the major contributor to this laxity. It can be repaired with a *plication of the posterior limb of the medial canthal tendon*. A conjunctival incision is made in the fold behind the caruncle, although some prefer to open the conjunctiva immediately behind the plica semilunaris. This incision is extended anteriorly to the medial end of the tarsal plate. A 00 lacrimal probe is placed in the lower canaliculus to be sure of its position at all times. Its tip is used to indicate the position of the lacrimal sac, making it easier to identify the posterior lacrimal crest. It is this area that is exposed to allow fixation of one end of a non-absorbable suture. The other end is secured in the

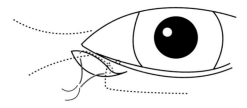

Figure 3.7 Medial canthal tendon plication – anterior limb.

posterior surface of the medial end of the tarsus, close to its superior border (Figure 3.8). The knot is buried and the conjunctiva closed.

Medial canthal resection is more appropriate if the punctum can be pulled laterally beyond the pupil. Here the horizontal shortening is medial as well as lateral to the punctum. A vertical incision is made perpendicular to the lid margin, just lateral to the caruncle. This of course necessitates cutting through the inferior canaliculus (Figure 3.9a). An 00

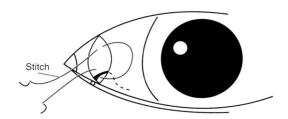

Figure 3.8 Medial canthal tendon plication – posterior limb.

lacrimal probe is maintained in the cut medial end of the canaliculus. As before, the tip of this probe can help in identifying the position of the posterior lacrimal crest. It is the periosteum just superior and posterior to this that is exposed with blunt dissection. The globe is kept safely lateral to the surgical site with small malleable retractors.

The degree of slack that can be taken up is measured by overlap until the lid margin is taut, as previously described. This portion is resected. A non-absorbable suture is placed as for posterior limb plication; however, before tying this, the cut medial end of the canaliculus is secured by marsupialisation and suturing to the top 1mm of the postero-medial corner of the newly shortened tarsus, with fine long-acting, absorbable sutures (Figure 3.9b). The skin closure is standard.

Total tarsal eversion

In this case the attachment of the lower lid retractors to the lower border of the tarsus is

lax. The inflammation and oedema of the exposed conjunctiva is often sufficient to maintain the lid in an everted position. This can occur unusually as an isolated incident,

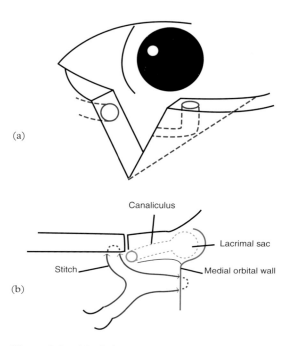

(a)

(b)

Figure 3.9 Medial canthal resection. (a) canaliculus cut, lid to be resected. (b) marsupialisation and reattachment of resected canaliculus.

where the possibility of a mechanical/cicatricial element has to be excluded. More usually, it presents as a long term result of untreated progressive ectropia. In these cases, surgical repair would therefore also need to include correction of whatever horizontal laxity was present.

Correction of the lower lid retractor laxity is achieved by *reattachment of the retractors to the inferior border of the tarsus*. A horizontal incision is made along the inferior tarsal border and the lower lid retractors identified. These can be resutured to the tarsal border as part of the conjunctival closure.

Inverting sutures raise the anterior lamella relative to the posterior lamella and are very useful when the chronically exposed conjunctiva is in the way of proper apposition of the lid to the globe, once the ectropion repair has been otherwise correctly completed. The redundant oedematous conjunctiva can be stretched inferiorly and kept in that position by long acting absorbable sutures pulled through from the anterior surface of the fornix to the skin. The track of the sutures should run inferiorly and anteriorly so they exit at the skin surface at the level of the inferior orbital rim (Figure 3.10). Here the sutures are tied over small bolsters, and can be removed after 14 days if they have not already fallen out.

It is not usually necessary to excise the redundant conjunctiva. However, if its bulk is such as to prevent correct apposition of the eyelid to the globe at the end of appropriately carried out surgery, even with the help of inverting sutures, then some of the conjunctiva can be sacrificed.

Inverting sutures may also be used as a temporary measure to control an ectropion, while waiting for definitive surgery.

Mechanical ectropion

If a growth or a cyst is responsible for pulling the lid margin down, it should be excised as vertically as possible. This will avoid a cicatricial ectropion. If the lesion has caused

horizontal laxity, this should be surgically corrected at the same time.

Cicatricial ectropion

A variety of conditions, congenital and acquired, result in skin shortage which pulls the lid margin away from the globe. Both lids may be affected, and the skin shortage causing the failure of normal lid closure may be localised or diffuse.

The assessment and management of cicatricial ectropion is covered in Chapter 2. However it is worth emphasising that skin shortage can be present with lid margin laxity. When the skin shortage is surgically repaired, the horizontal laxity needs to be corrected as well to prevent recurrence of the lid malposition.

Paralytic ectropion

The failure of lid closure in this situation is due to seventh nerve palsy. Correction requires both support and lid tightening procedures. The ectropion may have been present long enough to be associated with skin shrinkage. All these aspects of facial palsy are covered in Chapter 7.

Complications

Wound dehiscence and infection are unusual with careful surgery and aseptic techniques, but still occur with the latter commonly being the cause of the former. Wound dehiscence in the absence of infection is more likely to be iatrogenic and due to poor apposition of edges, lack of attention to anatomical layers, and sloppy knot tying.

Bruising is an expected side effect of surgery particularly in elderly patients, who form the great majority of those undergoing ectropion surgery. Nevertheless they should be warned of this. Unless of vital medical importance, chronic daily use of aspirin should be stopped a minimum of 10 days prior to surgery to allow platelet aggregation some recovery.

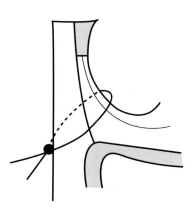

Figure 3.10   Inverting sutures.

Patients on anticoagulants, such as warfarin, should avoid lid surgery if the International Normalised Ratio (INR) cannot be brought down to between 2 and 2·2.

Haemorrhage tracking into the orbital cavity, to the extent of raising intraorbital pressure and potentially causing blindness secondary to optic nerve compression, is rare but a well recognised complication of lateral canthal tendon surgery in particular. It is best avoided by ensuring that the surgical site is absolutely dry prior to closure. If the patient exhibits the above symptoms, the lateral canthal corner is reopened as a matter of emergency to allow the sequestrated blood out, thereby relieving the pressure.

Ectropion repair hopefully results in long term success. However it is known that *recurrent ectropion* occurs in some 10% of patients in the three years following surgery. More often than not this is due to an underestimation of the horizontal shortening required: the repaired lid should be sufficiently taut at the end of surgery to just allow the closed tips of a small blunt instrument, such as a Barraquer needle holder, under the lid margin.

Recurrent ectropia should be assessed as if new and the anatomical cause addressed. A pentagon excision will usually correct any laxity. If the remnant laxity is in the canthal tendons, either because they were not accurately assessed preoperatively or because they became lax subsequently over time, then canthal tendon surgery is more appropriate than a pentagon excision.

Ectropion consecutive to entropion surgery is usually as a result of either undercorrection of lid laxity (corrected as indicated above) or due to overzealous reattachment or plication of the retractors. If tarsal eversion is obvious at the time of surgery or immediately afterwards, it is advisable to relax/replace the sutures attaching the retractors to the tarsus. If the ectropion becomes evident later, such as a week post operatively, the lid should be massaged with a clean finger very slightly greased with antibiotic ointment, several times a day until the lid resumes a normal position. If this has not been achieved over 8 to 12 weeks, the lower lid retractors will need to be released and reattached to the tarsus, but on hang back sutures. If the ectropion is as a result of too aggressive a removal of skin resulting in shortage, this will need to be replaced with a graft.

Consecutive entropion following ectropion surgery is unusual. Some internal marginal rotation, rather than frank entropion, may be noted during surgery: this is not uncommon particularly in the reattachment of canthal tendons to periosteum. This rotation is caused by the needle entries in the periosteum not being mirrored by the direction of entry in the new tarsal edge. This is corrected by resiting of the suture at the time of surgery, rather than hoping it will "settle down" into the right position. Entropion as a long term complication of ectropion repair is often associated with orbicularis override, and is treated accordingly.

An aggressive resection of the conjunctiva when repairing the laxity of the capsulo-palpebral attachment of the lower lid retractors will shorten the posterior lamella and result in the equivalent of a *cicatricial entropion*. This is best corrected with a mucous membrane graft to restore fornix depth. If the lid is still lax and there is excess lid skin, some may advocate the easier to perform lateral canthal strip procedure and blepharoplasty; however this alone does not address the loss of fornix depth.

Plication of the anterior limb of the medial canthal tendon can result in *antero-displacement of the canthal corner* if the medial canthal stitch is not placed superiorly and posteriorly to the stitch in the tarsus. This is best corrected at the time of surgery, but can be performed at a later date if the anteroposition has not been noticed at the time of the original operation.

Involutional ectropion is not a pathological entity but a result of becoming less young. Therefore it is not possible to promise a patient that surgery will guarantee a permanent cure: as long as the ageing process continues so will tissue degeneration. Nevertheless, an accurate preoperative assessment of the various factors contributing to the lid malposition, together with an appropriate combination of procedures as outlined above, are likely to result in success.

Further reading

Anderson RL, Gordy DD. The tarsal strip procedure. *Arch Ophthalmol* 1979;**97**:219–26.

Bick MW. Surgical management of orbital tarsal disparity. *Arch Ophthalmol* 1966;**75**:386–9.

Danks JJ, Rose GE. Involutional lower lid entropion: to shorten or not to shorten? *Ophthalmology* 1998;**105**: 2065–7.

Jones LT. An anatomical approach to problems of the eyelids and lacrimal apparatus. *Arch Ophthalmol* 1961; **66**:137–50.

McCord CD. Canalicular resection with canaliculostomy. *Ophthalmic Surg* 1980;**11**:440–5.

Smith BC. 'Lazy T' operation for the correction of ectropion. *Arch Ophthalmol* 1976;**90**:1149–50.

Tenzel RR, Buffam FV, Miller GR. The use of the lateral canthal sling in ectropion repair. *Can J Ophthalmol* 1977; **12**:199–202.

Tse DT, Kronish JW, Buus D. Surgical correction of lower eyelid ectropion by reinsertion of retractors. *Arch Ophthalmol* 1991;**109**:427–31.

4 Entropion

Ewan G Kemp

Entropion refers to any form of inverted lid margin.

The normal physiological position of the upper and lower eyelid margin is dependent on the relationship between the anterior and posterior lid lamellae (Figures 4.1 and 4.2). These are tightly bound together at the lid margin but elsewhere slippage can occur to cause either an entropion or ectropion. The lamella structure of the lids imparts rigidity and movement which has been well documented by Mustarde. The lids are opened by the lid retractors. In the upper lid these are mainly the levator muscle with its aponeurosis and Müller's muscle. In the lower lid they are fascial expansions from the inferior rectus muscle with some associated slips of smooth muscle. The lids are closed by the palpebral orbicularis muscle (Figure 4.3). In involutional entropion all the tissues become lax. In the lower lid, the retractors no longer hold the lower border of the tarsus downwards. The fascial extensions which form the skin crease become lax allowing the pre-septal muscle to move upwards over the pre-tarsal muscle and the lid inverts. In the upper lid, laxity leads to some sagging of the anterior lamella with reduction of the skin crease. The increased size of the tarsus gives more stability and the lid margin rarely inverts.

The stability of the lid margin is dependent on the interdigitation of the cilia, connective tissue and the muscle of Riolan on the anterior part of the terminal tarsus. The

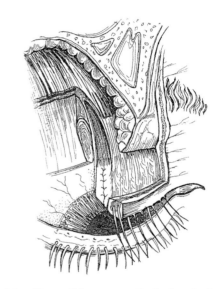

Figure 4.1   Upper lid anatomy displaying the lamella structure.

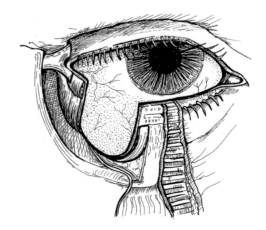

Figure 4.2   Lower lid anatomy displaying lower lid retractor complex.

24

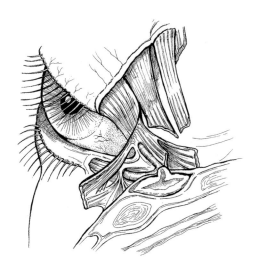

Figure 4.3   The orbicularis muscle, medial canthal anatomy and lacrimal canaliculi.

orifices of between 25 and 35 meibomian lands open on the upper lid margin compared to between 15 and 25 in the lower lid. These glands produce the oily layer of the tear film. The lash follicles also have smaller glands: the glands of Zeiss which are sebaceous, and the glands of Moll which are apocrine. They both deposit their fluid directly into the lash follicles. In entropion not only lashes abraid the cornea but undiluted secretion from the tarsal plate glands also cause irritation. If the keratinising process present at the mouths of the glands increases through disease it can cause a physical corneal abrasion. The hostile corneal environment is initially visible as a superficial punctate keratitis, which if allowed to progress will cause a full-thickness stromal defect which can perforate or scar.

Entropion is classified as:

- Involutional
- Congenital
- Cicatricial
- Spastic

Involutional entropion

The primary object of treatment is to rotate the lashes and lid margin away from the cornea and to prevent slippage between the lamellae. This is most easily achieved by placing everting sutures. In the lower lid these are placed through the lid from the conjunctival fornix to skin. In the upper lid because of potential corneal abrasion the sutures must remain on the anterior surface of the tarsal plate. They must elevate the skin and orbicularis muscle and hold them at a higher level on the tarsus, thus everting the lashes. The simplest method is often short-lived and patients therefore have to be warned that more complicated procedures may be required in the future should there be a subsequent failure. If more complicated pathology exists then more extensive procedures have to be adopted (Figures 4.4 and 4.5).

Congenital entropion

Congenital entropion is a relatively rare but usually benign condition. Surgical intervention requires to be modified for each case. Epiblepharon is more common and is present more frequently in the oriental races. Due to a variation in septal configuration and overall smaller orbital dimensions, the oriental lid displays overridings of the posterior lamella by a roll of skin and preseptal orbicularis. Time is often all that is needed to secure the integrity of the cornea as initially the lashes are soft and nonabrasive, only causing symptoms when the child matures. However if the cornea is compromised and the child is symptomatic the excision of the excess tissue of the anterior lamella is necessary. A horizontal section of anterior lamella is removed from the area anterior to the tarsal plate. Approximate measurements are taken and the wound is closed using a suture that tracks from the skin surface deep to the tarsal plate and back up to the skin surface. The mere closure of this wound everts the lid. If insufficient tissue has been removed the lid will not evert properly and further excision is required.

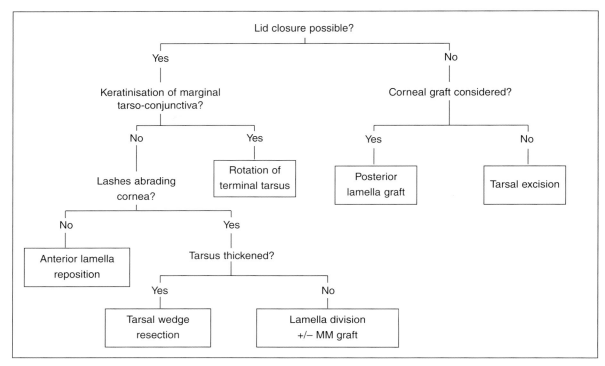

Figure 4.4   System for upper lid entropion. From: *A Manual of Systematic Eyelid Surgery* (2nd Edition), Churchill Livingstone, 1989.

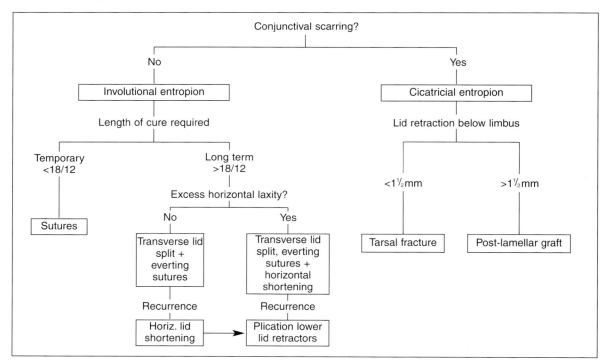

Figure 4.5   System for acquired lower lid entropion. From: *A Manual of Systematic Eyelid Surgery* (2nd Edition), Churchill Livingstone, 1989.

Cicatricial entropion

Cicatricial entropion causes misdirection of lashes when shortening of the posterior lamella follows contraction of scar tissue. The underlying pathology can vary and includes infection (trachoma chlamydia, chronic blepharoconjunctivitis and Herpes Zoster Ophthalmicus), toxic epithelial necrolysis (Stevens-Johnson syndrome), pemphigoid and trauma (chemical, thermal and mechanical). Histology is sometimes required to determine the nature of the condition.

Repair of these conditions not only includes rotation of the lid margin but modification or the addition of material to the foreshortened posterior lamella. Replacing like with like is a standard maxim so the posterior lamella requires replacement with tarsoconjunctiva if at all possible. When this is not readily available various auto-, homo- and allografts may be used, which all attempt to lengthen the tarsoconjunctival surface and allow the lashes to point away from the globe. The upper lid graft has one main objective and that is to maintain a moist surface in contact with the cornea. Gravity and muscle dynamics keep the tissues in contact. The lower lid, which works against gravity, requires a more rigid scaffold to support the skin and mucosal surface against the cornea. Material can be harvested from various sites and includes hard palate mucosa, nasal septal cartilage and ear cartilage. This requires a separate mucosal lining in order to protect the eye. Hard palate mucosa that has sufficient collagen matrix to remain rigid is probably the best form of substitute that can be adapted for both the lower and upper lid if tarsoconjunctival tissue is unavailable.

Spastic entropion

Spastic entropion occurs as a primary event in essential blepharospasm. It is a term that is often incorrectly used to describe the overriding of the tarsal plate by preseptal orbicularis which causes corneal irritation and secondary muscle spasm. Correction of any lid laxity and repair of the loss of contact between lid retractors, tarsal plate and skin is all that is usually required. If there is a primary spastic problem, then use of botulinum toxin is a possible temporary measure to be followed by limited excision of orbicularis oculi if a more permanent solution is required. Involutional entropion, often incorrectly termed spastic, is dependent on ageing change allowing tone to relax in the retractors and orbicularis muscles. Canthal ligaments stretch and the tarsal plates develop a less rigid structure with the deposit of more elastin. The sheer size of the tarsal plate is thought to determine whether the tarsus everts or inverts in such circumstances.

Surgical techniques

Surgical principles are dictated by clinical presentation and underlying pathology. Lax lids require increase in tone, canthal ligaments may require shortening and tarsal plates may need support. Lid retractors have to be reconnected to the tarsus and various combinations of technique can be adopted to suit most circumstances.

Surgery for lower lid

- Everting sutures
- Wies procedure
- Quickert procedure
- Jones procedure
- Tarsal dissection +/− mucous membrane grafting.

Everting sutures

For the most benign form of entropion where there is incompetence of the lid retractors, all that is required are everting sutures. These can be 4/0 catgut double-armed sutures. It is possible to gain a similar

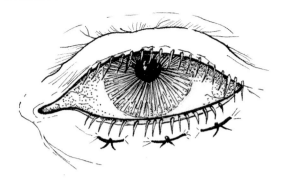

Figure 4.6   Everting sutures for lower lid entropion.

effect using 6/0 gauge sutures. Three sutures per lid are average (Figure 4.6). Care must be taken that the most medial suture is not over tightened as this may well cause punctal ectropion, creating epiphora where none existed before. Excessive secondary ectropion causing excessive exposure of the conjunctiva allows secondary keratinisation of the epithelium.

The ideal position post operatively is a lid margin which approximates the cornea. The sutures should create a deep crease on downgaze indicating that the lid retractors have been re-attached to the anterior lamella. Everting sutures, although used alone, can also be part of more elaborate procedures. If they are used alone the effect can only be guaranteed for about eighteen months to two years. Should the lid display not only incompetence of lid retractors but laxity at canthal ligaments or even distortion of the tarsal plate, then further surgery is required concentrating on these main areas. Distortion of the tarsal plate will require either direct shortening or dissection of excessive fibrosis. Laxity of the canthal ligaments requires some form of support or excision and shortening of the tissue, particularly at the junction between canthal ligament and tarsal plate. Care must be taken not to excessively shorten the lid or canthal ligaments, as this will prevent the lid from rising to its normal level and may well create a degree of overexposure of the inferior

corneal limbus. Specific procedures that incorporate these principles for the lower lid are as follows:

Wies procedure

A transverse skin incision is made below the level of the proximal margin of the tarsal plate and carried through into the fornix. The lid retractors are then identified and directly sutured from the lower fornix up the front of the tarsal plate and tied across the skin 2mm below the lash margin. This creates a fibrous barrier to any inappropriate action of anterior lamella across the posterior, thus stopping inversion of the lid margin. The traction sutures through to the skin keep the lid everted. The skin wound can be approximated with three or four 6/0 silk or nylon sutures.

Quickert's procedure

Quickert's procedure is a more complicated surgical undertaking. The Wies operation is combined with horizontal lid shortening. A Wies type transverse blepharotomy incision is made. A section of full thickness lid is excised and the free edges approximated while the lower lid retractors are brought through to the skin in a similar fashion to the Wies procedure. Any relative excess of skin and orbicularis muscle below the transverse skin wound can be excised.

Jones procedure

The lower lid retractors are plicated. A transverse lid incision is made through skin and orbicularis to expose the lower lid retractors. This layer is dissected and shortened with sutures which connect it to the proximal margin of the tarsal plate. As the wound is resutured the deep layers are connected through to the skin. This is only going to be a success when there is little or no horizontal lid laxity; additional lid shortening is necessary if this feature is present.

Tarsal dissection +/− mucous membrane grafting

The treatment of a cicitricial lower lid entropion depends on the degree of shortening of the posterior lamella and the lid retraction this has caused. If this is relatively minor the tarsus can be cut transversely and three or four double armed everting sutures passed from below the inferior tarsal margin to exit just below the lash line. When these sutures are tied on the skin the cut tarsus is hinged into eversion. The wound in the tarsus is allowed to granulate.

If the lid retraction is more marked a graft is required to lengthen the posterior lamella. The tarsus is cut transversely in exactly the same way and the graft sutured into the wound. The everting sutures are placed through the graft to hold it against its bed of pretarsal orbicularis muscle. They exit the skin just below the lash line and are tied sufficiently tightly to gently evert the lid margin.

Surgery for upper lid

- Anterior lamella repositioning with everting sutures
- Tarsal margin split
- Posterior lamella advance following lid split
- Distal margin rotation +/− mucous membrane grafting.

Anterior lamella repositioning with everting sutures

If the upper lid entropion is mild, the anterior lamella can be elevated and held in position with everting sutures. A skin crease incision is made. The anterior tarsal surface is dissected to the lash roots. Everting or repositioning sutures are passed from high on the tarsus and exit the skin just above the eyelashes where they are tied to give gentle eyelash eversion. The skin crease is reformed.

Tarsal margin split

If the eversion of the lid margin is insufficient with an anterior lamella repositioning type of procedure, it can be increased by splitting the grey line to a depth of about 2mm. The incision should be just posterior to the lash follicles and the open wound heals by granulation.

Posterior lamella advance following lid split

Lid retraction in the upper lid can be managed by recessing the upper lid retractors or adding a posterior lamella graft. If the retraction is mild the posterior lamella of the eyelid can be advanced by totally freeing Müller's muscle and all the scar tissues under the conjunctiva. This can be done as part of an anterior lamella repositioning procedure with or without a grey line split, or more specifically as a procedure on its own. A grey line split is extended up onto the anterior surface of the tarsus and continued to totally free the posterior lamella from all tissue to the upper fornix. The lid lamellae are then held together with sutures that are passed from the fornix directly through to the skin. The terminal anterior surface of the advanced tarsus is left bare to granulate and the lid margin sutured directly to it (Figure 4.7).

Distal margin rotation +/− mucous membrane grafting

If lid retraction is more severe the posterior lamella may need to be lengthened with a graft. Hard palate mucosa (Figure 4.8) is preferable as it is stiffer than labial or buccal mucosa and is wettable. Nasal septal cartilage with its mucoperichondrium is an alternative. The upper tarsus can be incised transversely and the graft inserted between the cut edges as for a lower lid cicitricial entropion repair. The terminal tarsus usually needs to be

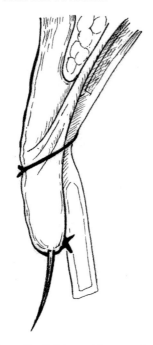

Figure 4.7   Lamella division with posterior advance.

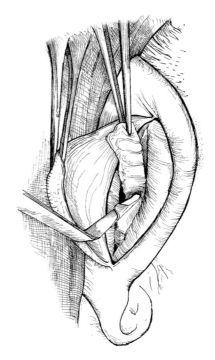

Figure 4.9   Ear cartilage harvest for entropion repair.

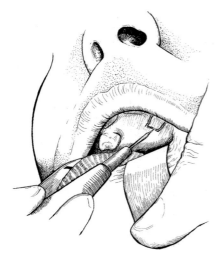

Figure 4.8   Hard palate harvest for posterior lamella graft.

rotated away from the globe. Any keratinised epithelium in contact with the cornea should be excised.

Ear cartilage (Figure 4.9) is not good as a posterior lamella graft in the upper lid as it causes corneal irritation if it is not covered by conjunctiva or mucosa. Its main use in upper lid entropion surgery is as a sandwich graft to stiffen the reconstructed lid which has, for instance, been made up from skin and mucosa. The insertion of the ear cartilage between these two lamellae will allow the lid margin to be everted satisfactorily.

Trichiasis

Trichiasis is the term used for distorted eyelashes. They may arise from a normal position i.e. from lash roots that are just anterior to the tarsal plate (aberrant eyelashes) or from an abnormal position (dysplastic eyelashes). Blepharitis and chronic external eye disease are the commonest causes of aberrant eyelashes, but anything which leads to scarring of the lid margin can be responsible e.g. trauma. Dysplastic lashes are caused by chronic ongoing external eye disease conditions such as pemphigoid which may lead to eyelashes arising from the posterior lid margin.

If the lid margin position is abnormal, this must first be corrected as described in this chapter. If the eyelashes themselves are abnormal they must be destroyed. Various methods have been described including electrolysis, cryotherapy, laser etc.

Electrolysis

This is the treatment of choice for one, two or very few aberrant eyelashes. The disadvantage is the difficulty of inserting the needle accurately down the hair follicle to the root. If it comes out of the follicle it causes collateral damage which in its turn creates more scarring and further trichiasis.

Cryotherapy

This is the standard treatment for more than a very few lashes. The lash follicles are sensitive to cold and are destroyed by a temperature of $-20°C$. The destructive effect is more marked if a double freeze-thaw cycle is applied. The disadvantage is that all the lashes exposed to cryotherapy are destroyed and it can cause depigmentation as melanocyte, are sensitive to $-10°C$. This means they are destroyed before the temperature is cold enough to destroy the lash roots.

Distichiasis

This is the condition in which a second row of eyelashes grow out of the Meibomian gland orifices. It can be treated by electrolysis, but there is a high failure or recurrence rate. If the lid is split into two lamellae with an extended grey line split (*vide supra*), the terminal posterior lamella can be treated with cryotherapy. The lid can then be reconstituted with sutures leaving the posterior lamella a little proud to allow for any shrinkage after the freezing.

An alternative treatment for distichiasis is to evert the lid and cut the tarsus following the course of each involved eyelash to its root. This can then be treated under direct vision with cautery or electrolysis. The disadvantage of this is the time that it takes, but it can be a very effective treatment.

Further reading

Collin JRO. Congenital entropion. In: *A Manual of Systematic Eyelid Surgery* (2nd ed). London: Churchill Livingstone, 1989: 14.

El-Mulki S, Lawson J, Taylor D. A new and simple procedure for correction of congenital tarsal kink. *J Pediatr Ophthalmol Strabismus* 1991; **35**:172–3.

Jones LT, Reeh MJ, Wobig JL. Senile entropion – a new concept for correction. *Am J Ophthalmol* 1972; **74**:327.

Kemp EG, Collin JRO. Surgical management of upper lid entropion. B J Ophthalmol 1986; **20**:575–9.

Liu D. Lower eyelid tightening: A comparative study. *Ophthal Plas Reconstr Surg* 1997; **13**:199–203.

Mustarde J. Reconstruction of the upper lid. In: *Repair and Construction of the Orbital Region* (3rd ed). Edinburgh: Churchill Livingstone, 1991: 191.

Quickert MH, Rathburn JE. Suture repair of entropion. *Arch Ophthalmol* 1971; **85**:304.

Shorlin JP, Lemke BN. Clinical eyelid anatomy. In: Bosniak S, ed. *Principles and Practices of Ophthalmic Plastic and Reconstructive Surgery*. Vol 1. (1st Edition). London: W B Saunders Company, 1996: 261.

Steel EHW, Hoh HB, Harrad R, Collins CR. Botulinum toxin for the temporary treatment of involutional lower lid entropion: A clinical and morphological study. *Eye* 1997; **11**:472–5.

Trabut G. Entropion – trichiasis en afrique du nord. *Arch d'Ophthalmologie* 1949; **9**:701.

Tyers AG, Collin JRO. Involutional entropion In: *Colour Atlas of Ophthalmic Plastic Surgery* (1st Edition). Oxford: Butterworth Heinemann, 1995: 69.

Yang LLH, Lambert S, Chapman J, Stulting RD. Congenital entropion and congenital cornea ulcer. *Am J Ophthalmol* 1996; **121**:329–31.

Yaqub A, Leatherbarrow B. The use of autogenous auricular cartilage in the management of upper eyelid entropion. *Eye* 1997; **1**:801–5.

Wies F. Spastic entropion. *Trans Am Acad Ophthalmol Otolaryngol* 1955; **59**:503.

5 Ptosis

Ruth Manners

Blepharoptosis describes a drooping of the upper eyelid and is derived from the Greek words **blepharon** = eyelid and **ptosis** = falling down. The term is almost invariably abbreviated to ptosis.

Assessment of ptosis

There are many features, both ophthalmic and systemic, which need to be assessed to elucidate the cause of ptosis and plan management:

History

The history should include the following information: age of onset, family history, past ocular history (including previous intraocular or lid surgery), predisposing factors such as contact lens wear or trauma, episodes of lid swelling, whether the ptosis worsens throughout the day, the presence of any aberrant lid movements, whether eye movements are impaired and if there is diplopia. The past medical history and current medications are also important when planning surgery.

Palpebral aperture (PA)

With the eyes in primary position the widest distance between the upper and lower lid margins is measured in millimetres with a transparent ruler held directly in front of the lids (Fig. 5.1a). It is important to ensure there is no

frontalis overaction. Drawings and photographs are often the easiest method of describing contour abnormalities, scleral show etc.

Margin-reflex distance (MRD)

Since palpebral aperture is not only affected by the degree of ptosis but also by the lower lid position (Figure 5.1b), it is sometimes more useful to get the patient to fixate a point light source in the primary position and to measure the distance from the corneal light

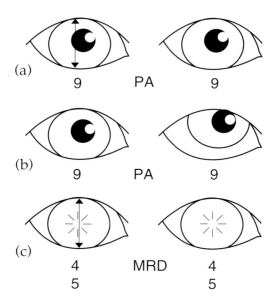

Figure 5.1   Palpebral aperture measurement.
(a) Vertical measurement.
(b) Same vertical measurement with left ptosis compensated by left lower lid retraction.
(c) Margin reflex distance measurement.

reflex to the upper lid margin (MRD1) and from the reflex to the lower lid margin (MRD2) (Figure 5.1c).

The two numbers are recorded thus

4	MRD 1	3
5	MRD 2	5

The upper lid may obscure the visual axis in which case MRD 1 is recorded as a negative number.

Accentuation

In any unilateral ptosis, but especially in acquired aponeurotic ptosis, an underlying asymmetrical bilateral ptosis may be present. The voluntary effort required to lift the more ptotic lid is associated with increased innervation to the less ptotic lid due to Hering's law, which may normalise its position. The patient is asked to maintain primary position without blinking and the ptotic lid manually lifted by the examiner. The "normal" lid is examined to see whether it shows a gradual droop once the excess drive to its levator is removed.

Levator function (LF)

A measurement of eyelid excursion from extreme upgaze to extreme downgaze is recorded in millimetres which gives an estimate of levator function (although true muscle function i.e. force, is not actually being measured). To eradicate the accessory elevatory input of frontalis muscle, it should be splinted against the forehead with a thumb. Normal levator function is about 15mm or more. It is arbitrarily divided into three grades: good >10mm, moderate, 5–10mm and poor <5mm and is the most important factor in deciding on the type of surgery required.

Skin crease (SC)

The anatomical distance from the upper lid margin to the eyelid crease is measured with the patient looking down (Figure 5.2). There

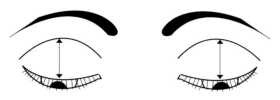

Figure 5.2   Skin crease measurement.

may be more than one skin crease but generally there is a dominant one which becomes apparent when the patient moves their lid. Excess upper lid skin may overhang the skin crease and should be gently lifted out of the way, without stretching the skin, to enable the skin crease to be measured.

In the primary position, the distance from the lid margin to the edge of the overhanging upper lid skin is known as the pretarsal show and is an important cosmetic aspect. It is affected both by the skin crease position and the lid position.

Pupil size

Miosis in Horner's syndrome will be seen on the affected side and can be confirmed with the Cocaine 4% test. Mydriasis may be present in a third nerve palsy.

Cover test

It is imperative to exclude hypotropia and pseudoptosis. In about 30% of children with ptosis there is co-existant strabismus and if strabismus surgery is planned, it should be performed prior to ptosis repair.

Extraocular muscle function

Extraocular movements may be diminished in many conditions that cause ptosis such as third nerve palsy, myopathies, congenital ocular fibrosis syndrome and also in ptosis with associated superior rectus weakness.

There are several factors which need to be assessed in order to determine the risk of post operative corneal exposure:

1. Strength of eyelid closure

The strength of orbicularis oculi is measured to assess the risk of post operative lagophthalmos and corneal exposure. The patient is asked to screw their eyes shut and on normal forced lid closure the eyelashes should be buried.

2. Bell's phenomenon

The patient closes his/her eyes whilst the examiner gently opens the lids to assess whether Bell's phenomenon is present or absent.

3. Lagophthalmos

Lagophthalmos may be present preoperatively and the amount should be measured. Parents and patients should be warned that levator surgery will probably exacerbate the degree of lagophthalmos.

4. Tear film assessment

A dry eye condition will put the patient at risk of corneal problems post operatively if any lagophthalmos is created.

5. Corneal sensation

This should be assessed prior to instillation of any anaesthetic drops.

Aberrant/synkinetic lid movements

Most aberrant movements will already be noted by the parents or patient. The relative importance of the aberrant movements and the ptosis should be ascertained in order to plan surgery. A jaw-wink can be demonstrated by asking the patient to open and close his/her mouth, to chew or to thrust the jaw from side to side.

Fatiguability

If there is a history of fatiguability of the lid, this should be tested. The patient is asked to maintain fixation on a target on the ceiling, without blinking, for as long as possible. However, after about 20 seconds, this is an extremely uncomfortable manouevre for anyone and therefore anaesthetic drops should be inserted in both eyes prior to the test. In myasthenia the ptosis will be seen to worsen.

Vision and refraction

In young children with ptosis, it is important to ensure that there is normal visual development in the affected eye(s). Occlusion amblyopia can occur due to severe ptosis but amblyopia more commonly results from associated strabismus or anisometropia. Vision and refraction should be measured regularly in children and treatment such as occlusion therapy, glasses, strabismus surgery or early ptosis surgery performed as appropriate.

Visual fields

Visual field assessment may help assess the degree of functional disturbance in adults with ptosis. Superior visual field loss is common when visual fields are measured with eyes in the primary position.

Compensatory head posture

A chin-up head posture can also represent a functional handicap to the patient by causing loss of balance or neck ache. In young children it may indicate that binocular vision is present but in severe cases this can hinder the child's motor development by delaying walking.

Frontalis action

Frontalis overaction may mask ptosis to some degree and it is important to be aware of this when assessing patients. When considering a brow suspension procedure it is necessary to check that good frontalis action is present. A point on the brow is defined and its excursion measured with the brow relaxed and then raised, which should be about 10mm (Figure 5.3). If the patient finds it difficult to relax a habitually raised brow then he/she should be instructed to frown and then relax.

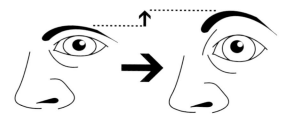

Figure 5.3   Measurement of frontalis action.

Lid position on downgaze

Note the lid position on downgaze; in aponeurotic ptosis it remains ptotic and in marked congenital myogenic ptosis it lags behind the normal lid.

Phenylephrine test

Three drops of 2·5% phenylephrine are instilled over a 10 minute period. This stimulates sympathetically innervated Müller's muscle and the degree of lid elevation after 15 minutes will help determine how the ptosis will respond to Müller's muscle surgery.

Ocular examination

A general ocular examination should also be performed looking for specific features associated with ptosis such as cataract, pigmentary retinopathy, etc.

Classification of ptosis

A mechanistic classification divides ptosis into different aetiological groups: myogenic, aponeurotic, neurogenic and mechanical. Within each group the ptosis may be congenital or acquired.

Myogenic

Due to a defect in the levator muscle.

Congenital myogenic (dysgenetic) ptosis

Congenital myogenic ptosis is a sporadic or more rarely inherited dysgenesis of the levator muscle resulting in reduced levator function and ptosis, either unilateral or bilateral.

The levator function varies from good to poor and similarly the ptosis ranges from mild to severe. When levator function is poor there is also lack of a skin crease and lag of the lid on downgaze since the muscle both contracts and relaxes inadequately. Lagophthalmos may also be present.

The initial priority is to assess the child's visual development and to treat any co-existant strabismus, ametropia and amblyopia. When severe unilateral ptosis covers the visual axis there is a risk of occlusion amblyopia and ptosis repair is required urgently. Similarly, bilateral ptosis with a marked chin-up head posture may require early intervention. If visual development is normal then most surgeons would delay surgery to about 4 years of age when more accurate pre-operative measurements are possible, and yet is prior to school age. The choice between levator resection and brow suspension depends on the levator function.

Blepharophimosis syndrome

Blepharophimosis syndrome is an autosomal dominant, inherited syndrome (gene on chromosome 3). Occasionally sporadic.

A combination of features are seen bilaterally including phimosis on the palpebral aperture, telecanthus, epicanthus inversus, ptosis with poor levator function and cicatricial ectropion of the lateral part of the lower lid.

If surgery for telecanthus and epicanthus inversus is required it should be performed at about 3 years of age, prior to ptosis surgery. A Y-V plasty with shortening of the underlying medial canthal tendon will correct the telecanthus and this is combined with double Z-plasties to overcome the vertical skin shortage causing the epicanthic folds. A combination of these two procedures results in Mustarde's "flying man" incision. Ptosis repair almost invariably requires brow suspension performed at about 5 years.

Myasthenia gravis

Autoimmune antibodies of unknown aetiology interrupt transmission of acetycholine at the neuro-muscular junctions of striated muscle by reducing available post-synaptic acetylcholine receptors causing fluctuating weakness of voluntary muscles.

The condition may be generalised or purely ocular. Bulbar muscle involvement causes difficulty in chewing and swallowing, skeletal muscle involvement causes weakness of movements and facial muscle involvement causes loss of facial expression. Ocular features include ophthalmoplegia of any type and ptosis which is the commonest presenting feature.

The Tensilon test identifies whether a dose of intravenous Tensilon (edrophonium hydrochloride) transiently improves an observable weakness such as ptosis. However, a negative result does not rule out myasthenia gravis. Serum antibodies to acetylcholine receptors are detectable in a majority but not all patients.

Medical treatment is with the use of long-acting anticholinesterase drugs. Systemic steroids and plasmapheresis are sometimes required. Some patients have a hyperplastic thymus and thymectomy may be useful.

Muscular dystrophy

This is a hereditary, progressive degeneration of muscle.

Myotonic dystrophy is an autosomal dominantly inherited muscular dystrophy showing the typical feature of myotonia i.e. persistant muscle contraction after a strong stimulation.

The ocular features include progressive bilateral ptosis, weakness of orbicularis oculi, strabismus, pre-senile cataracts, light-near dissociation and pigmentary retinopathy. Systemic features include myotonia of peripheral muscles and muscle wasting, expressionless facies with pre-frontal balding, respiratory weakness and cardiac hypertrophy.

The management is levator resection or brow suspension depending on the levator function. Ptosis repair needs to be cautious in view of the concomitant poor lid closure.

Oculopharyngeal dystrophy is an autosomal dominant condition (gene on chromosome 14). Characterised by ptosis with associated weakness of the pharyngeal muscles.

Mitochondrial myopathy is a primary muscle abnormality due to defective mitochondria. The mitochondrial myopathies are maternally inherited because mutated mitochondrial DNA is transmitted exclusively by the mother in the cytoplasm of the ovum.

It is characterised by bilateral progressive ptosis and chronic progressive external ophthalmoplegia (CPEO) which is often symmetrical and so does not give rise to diplopia. *Kearns Sayre syndrome* also shows pigmentary retinopathy and heart block. *MERRF* (Myoclonic Epilepsy and Ragged Red Fibres) has associated epilepsy and typical ragged red fibres of mitochondrial myopathy seen on Gomori trichrome staining of a muscle biopsy.

It is managed by cautious repair of ptosis with levator resection or brow suspension. General anaesthesia should be avoided in some of these patients because of the systemic features.

Congenital ocular fibrosis syndrome is an autosomal dominant condition (gene on chromosome 12) where the extraocular muscles show congenital fibrosis.

There is severe ptosis with poor levator function and a non-progressive external ophthalmoplegia where typically the extraocular movements are severely restricted and the eyes deviated downwards. On attempted upgaze the eyes converge. These features result in a marked chin-up compensatory head posture.

If the eyes are markedly deviated downwards then inferior rectus recessions or disinsertions may be required in the first instance. The ptosis requires brow suspension.

Other

Myogenic ptosis – may be due to:

- Trauma – levator function may continue to recover over a period of months: therefore ptosis surgery should be delayed for six months
- Post inflammation, for example, myositis
- Infiltration, for example, lymphoma.

Aponeurotic

Here there is a defect in the transmission of power from the levator muscle to the eyelid, due to stretching, dehiscence or disinsertion of the levator aponeurosis.

It may result from:

- Congenital – rare.
- Involutional – the commonest cause of ptosis. Often associated with other involutional changes in the peri-ocular tissues such as dermatochalasis, ectropion, entropion, brow ptosis and orbital fat prolapse.
- Trauma – may occur following blunt trauma and lid swelling or following intraocular surgery although the reasons for this are unclear. It can be related to contact lens wear and is thought to be due to repeated stretching of the lids on insertion of the lens. It can also occur as a sequel to the blepharochalasis syndrome.

The ptosis varies from mild to severe but levator function is always good. The skin crease is elevated or absent and the upper lid may be thinned with a deep upper lid sulcus. The ptotic eyelid remains ptotic in downgaze and consequently patients may complain of symptoms when reading.

Management requires reinsertion or tightening i.e. advancement or plication of the levator aponeurosis.

Neurogenic

Due to an innervational defect of levator palpebrae superioris or Müller's muscle.

Third nerve palsy

Posterior communicating artery aneurysm (especially if associated with pain), compressive lesion of the cavernous sinus, tumour, diabetes and ischaemia cause acquired oculomotor nerve palsies. Rarely the palsy is congenital.

The loss of levator function is proportional to the innervational defect and results in varying degrees of ptosis from mild to complete. The eye may be exotropic and hypotropic with poor Bell's phenomenon, all of which increase the risk of post operative corneal exposure. The pupil may be dilated especially in a "surgical" third nerve palsy e.g. due to an aneurysm. Other neurological deficits can also be present.

Many "medical" third nerve palsies recover within one to two months but if not, any co-existent squint needs to be dealt with initially. A levator resection or brow suspension is required depending on the levator function. Care is needed to avoid post operative lagophthalmos and subsequent corneal exposure.

Horner's syndrome

Results from an interruption of the sympathetic pathway somewhere along its long pathway. Lesions include carcinoma at the lung apex (Pancoast syndrome), lesions in the neck (trauma, surgery, malignant lymph nodes), internal carotid artery dissection and central nervous system lesions (demyelination, syringobulbia).

There is sympathetic denervation of Müller's muscle, its equivalent in the lower lid (inferior tarsal muscle) and sphincter pupillae. A mild ptosis of one to two millimetres results and the lower lid is minimally elevated. This change in the position of both lids gives the appearance of "apparent" enophthalmos even though the globe position is unchanged. Levator function is normal. Other features include miosis, heterochromia due to lack of iris pigmentation on the affected side if Horner's syndrome occurs congenitally or at a very young age, and anhydrosis if the lesion is below the superior cervical ganglion.

Diagnostic tests include:
- Cocaine (4%) test. One drop is placed in each eye. Over 30 minutes this prevents reuptake of noradrenaline at the neuromuscular synapse causing pupil dilation on the normal side but not on the affected side.
- Hydroxyamphetamine (1%) test (presently unavailable). One drop in each eye stimulates the release of noradrenaline from the postganglionic nerve ending and causes pupil dilatation in both eyes if the lesion is preganglionic but only on the normal side if the lesion is postganglionic.

The Fasanella-Servat procedure will treat the small degree of ptosis.

Marcus Gunn jaw-winking ptosis

Marcus Gunn jaw-winking ptosis is a developmental abnormality where the levator muscle co-contracts with stimulation of the trigeminal nerve supply to lateral pterygoid, medial pterygoid or both. Autosomal dominantly inherited or sporadic.

There is ptosis of varying severity with related degree of levator function often associated with superior rectus underaction. Movement of the jaw causes elevation of the upper lid i.e. the wink.

Abolition of the wink requires division of the levator muscle and subsequent brow suspension (unilateral, bilateral or levator transposition). Treatment of the ptosis alone should err towards undercorrection if there is a risk of post operatively accentuating the wink by exposing more sclera.

Aberrant regeneration of seventh nerve

Aberrant regeneration of seventh nerve may occur following a facial nerve palsy in which the lower branches of the nerve can grow to re-innervate orbicularis oculi resulting in ptosis with movement (or even resting tone) of the muscles of facial expression of the lower face. The ptosis which develops following a facial palsy; when the patient moves the lower facial muscles, for example, blows out the cheeks or simulates chewing, the upper lid droops. Abolition of the ptosis requires division of the levator muscle and brow suspension or levator transposition. The aberrant activity in the facial nerves may be reduced with cautious botulinum toxin injections to the orbicularis muscle.

Mechanical

Ptosis can occur due to excessive lid mass or bulk or to a scarring process in the lid.

It may result from:
- Lesions in the upper lid such as Meibomian cyst, haemangioma, plexiform neuroma of neurofibromatosis or malignant tumours for example, basal cell, squamous cell and Meibomian gland carcinomas.
- Cicatrising conditions in the lid such as conjunctival scarring.
- Trauma which can cause scarring in the lid which may act as a mass or as a splint causing mechanical ptosis.

Treatment is directed to the primary cause such as removal of a lid lump or scar mass or grafting to relieve cicatrised tissue.

Pseudoptosis

It is vitally important to exclude pseudoptosis on examination of the patient and the following causes should be borne in mind:

- Ipsilateral – Hypotropia, enophthalmos, dermatochalasis, brow ptosis and blepharospasm.
- Contralateral – Lid retraction, exophthalmos.

Surgical correction of ptosis

There is always some unpredictability in ptosis repair and thus there will always be a need for revision surgery in some patients. Post operative corneal protection is of paramount importance and this may influence the amount of ptosis surgery performed. The levator function is the essential determining factor in choosing the surgical procedure in ptosis repair.

Levator resection

Indications

Myogenic or neurogenic ptosis with moderate or good levator function i.e. 5mm or more, when the levator can be shortened to lift the lid. Levator resection will not be effective when levator function is poor i.e. 4mm or less.

Procedure (Figure 5.4)

The approach can be anteriorly through the intended skin crease position or posteriorly through the conjunctiva. The amount of levator resected is based on both the degree of ptosis and the levator function. The levator is identified and freed from underlying tissues and shortened by between 12 to 30mm. In larger resections the lateral and medial horns of the muscle are divided to allow the muscle to be advanced sufficiently. The resected muscle is then reattached with about three sutures to the anterior, superior surface of the tarsus. The skin crease is reformed by incorporating a bite of the lower edge of the levator muscle in the skin wound.

Internal Whitnall sling – Where there is marked ptosis and levator function is not good (5mm or less) the levator can be slung over Whitnall's ligament which acts as an internal suspension for the lid. This gives very little lid movement post operatively.

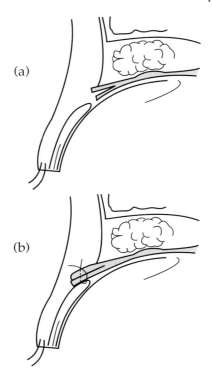

(a)

(b)

Figure 5.4 Anterior approach levator resection. The levator muscle is resected after excising the aponeurosis and Müller's muscle (a), and reopposed to tarsus (b).

Aponeurosis surgery

Indications

Good levator function and evidence of aponeurotic ptosis. The choice of approach and initial surgery are as for levator resections.

Procedure (Figure 5.5)

An anterior approach has the advantage that excess skin can be excised where patients have co-existing dermatochalasis. Sometimes a true disinsertion of the levator aponeurosis is identified and the lower edge of the aponeurosis can then be reinserted onto the tarsal plate. In aponeurosis stretching, the aponeurosis is advanced sufficiently to eradicate the ptosis. Since the vast majority of aponeurotic ptosis occurs in adults, this surgery should be performed under local

(a)

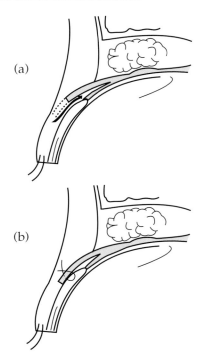

(b)

Figure 5.5 Aponeurosis advancement with direct sutures. Separated from underlying Müller's muscle (a), and advanced on to the tarsus (b).

anaesthesia so that perioperative adjustment of the lid height can be made.

Aponeurosis tuck (Figure 5.6) – some surgeons prefer not to free the aponeurosis from the underlying tissues but to merely plicate the tendon with one or more sutures.

Adjustable sutures (Figure 5.7) – to overcome some of the unpredictability of ptosis surgery, especially in patients undergoing redo surgery or in those adults who insist on surgery under general anaesthesia, adjustable sutures can be used to attach the levator muscle or aponeurosis to the tarsal plate. These can then be advanced or recessed within 24 hours following surgery.

Complications of levator resection and aponeurosis advancement

Overcorrections – if the lid is very high then immediate lowering is required. If the

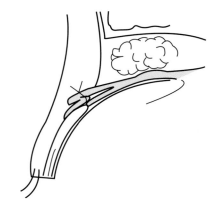

Figure 5.6 Aponeurosis tuck.

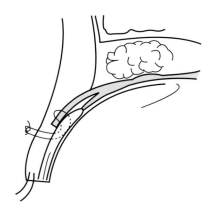

Figure 5.7 Aponeurosis advancement with adjustable sutures.

overcorrection is mild, instruct the patient to massage the lid with traction on the lashes regularly for up to three months. Wait six months and reassess.

Undercorrections – if marked, immediate re-do surgery is indicated. If mild, wait six months and review.

Abnormal contour – selective recession or advancement of the levator or aponeurosis.

Lagophthalmos and exposure – regular lubricant drops and ointment. Lowering the lid may be necessary if the cornea is jeopardised, requiring recession of the levator muscle.

Conjunctival prolapse – occurs more commonly with large levator resections if the suspensory ligament of the superior fornix is incised or prolapses. Copious lubricants should be given initially but if the prolapse does not settle after days to weeks then insert Pang-type sutures (full thickness sutures from superior fornix through the skin crease) or excise the prolapsed conjunctiva.

Lash ptosis – an inadequate skin crease requires reformation. However, if the skin crease is satisfactory, then an anterior lamella reposition is indicated.

Ectropion – this may occur if the levator is sutured too low onto the anterior surface of the tarsus or if placement of the sutures during skin crease reformation is too high. To correct the ectropion, the sutures need to be repositioned.

Brow suspension

Indications

Ptosis with poor or absent levator function i.e. 4mm or less, where an alternative source of power is required to lift the lid. The lid is therefore suspended to the frontalis muscle so that raising the brow also lifts the lid. This procedure can also be used following a levator division, undertaken to eradicate aberrant movements of the lid.

Procedure

The best suspensory material is autogenous fascia lata harvested from the thigh. Children under four years are generally too small to enable autogenous fascia lata to be used. Other autogenous materials include palmaris longus tendon and temporalis fascia. Non-autogenous materials are plentiful and all have the advantage of being easily available but their long term success rate is not as good as with autogenous fascia lata. Some non-autogenous materials include stored fascia (irradiated or lyophilised), Prolene, Supramid (polyfilament cable-type suture), Mersilene mesh, silicone cords (adjustable immediately post operatively when secured with a Watske sleeve), Gore-Tex (polytetrafluoroethylene, PTFE) and ePTFE (expanded PTFE).

Autogenous suspensory material is generally arranged as a double triangle (Crawford method – Figure 5.8a) thought to give a good lid contour whereas non-autogenous material is inserted as a pentagon (Fox method – Figure 5.8b) where less material is used and any subsequent Crawford brow suspension can be performed through uninvolved tissues. Brow suspension will only be effective if the patient uses frontalis muscle post operatively. If the ptosis is unilateral, some surgeons advocate division of the normal levator and bilateral brow suspension to gain greater symmetry. The options need to be discussed carefully with patients and their parents.

Levator transposition procedure – several surgeons advocate using the levator muscle itself as the suspensory material thus transposing the divided end of the muscle into the brow, eliminating the need for alternative suspensory material. In certain patients, neurotisation of the levator muscle from frontalis results in some post operative gain in levator function.

Complications of brow suspension

Overcorrection – release bands soon after initial surgery.

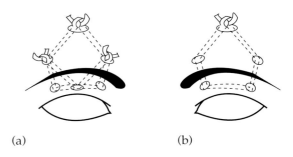

(a) (b)

Figure 5.8 Brow suspension – frontalis sling.
(a) Crawford technique.
(b) Fox pentagon.

Undercorrection – tighten bands in the early postoperative period. Redo surgery may ultimately be required. In mild cases a full thickness lid resection can be performed.

Exposure – lubricants initially but may ultimately require release of bands.

Late droop – redo brow suspension preferably with autogenous fascia lata to minimise risk of further late droop.

Infection/granulomas – systemic antibiotics and excision of granulomas.

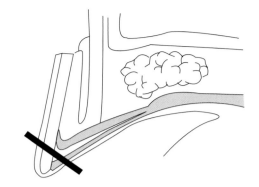

Figure 5.9   Cross-section showing tissue removed in Fasanella-Servat procedure.

Fasanella-Servat procedure (tarsomüllerectomy)

Indications

Small ptosis of 2mm or less with good levator function, for example Horner's syndrome.

Procedure (Figures 5.9 and 5.10)

The lid is everted and the upper border of the tarsus, together with the lower end of Müller's muscle and the conjunctiva, are held between clamps, excised and the free ends resutured. The main effect is thought to depend on the amount of tarsus excised. It is important to place the clamps correctly (Figure 5.10a) so that an equal amount of tissue is excised along the eyelid, and to avoid excess removal centrally by incorrect placement of the clamps (Figure 5.10b), which would result in a peaked lid. Some surgeons prefer to preserve the tarsus and suggest excising only Müller's muscle and conjunctiva to correct the ptosis.

Complications

Peaked lid – avoid by correct positioning of clamps on everted lid.

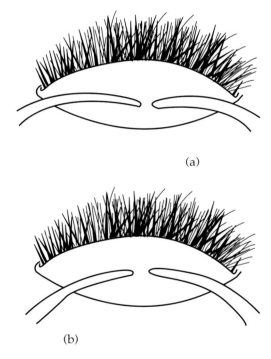

(a)

(b)

Figure 5.10   Fasanella-Servat procedure. Position of clamps, (a) correct; (b) incorrect.

Undercorrection – redo the procedure *if* the indications for surgery are correct i.e. minimal ptosis and good levator function.

Short tarsus – generally results from over zealous surgery for ptosis too severe to correct with a tarsomüllerectomy.

Corneal abrasion – insert a protective soft contact lens for a few weeks post operatively.

Ptosis props

Very occasionally ptosis props fixed to spectacles are indicated for patients with severe ptosis with both poor levator function and poor frontalis action. In general, patients will not tolerate ptosis props unless their orbicularis action is weak.

Further reading

Anderson RL, Dixon RS. Aponeurotic ptosis surgery. *Arch Ophthalmol* 1979; **97**:1123–8.

Beard C. Complications of ptosis surgery. *Ann Ophthalmol* 1972; **4**:671–5.

Berke RN, Wadsworth JAC. Histology of levator muscle in congenital and acquired ptosis. *Arch Ophthalmol* 1955; **53**:413–28.

Collin JRO. *A manual of systematic eyelid surgery* (2nd Edition). London: Churchill Livingstone, 1989.

Collin JRO, Beard C, Wood I. Experimental clinical data on the insertion of the levator palpebrae superioris muscle. *Am J Ophthalmol* 1978; **85**:792–801.

Collin JRO, O'Donnell BA. Adjustable sutures in eyelid surgery for ptosis and lid retraction. *Br J Ophthal* 1994; **78**:167–74.

Crawford JS. Repair of ptosis using frontalis and fascia lata. A 20 year review. *Ophthalmic Surg* 1977; **8**:31–40.

Dortzbach RK, Sutula FC. Involutional blepharoptosis – a histopathological study. *Arch Ophthalmol* 1980; **98**:1045–9.

Dryden RM, Fleming JC, Quickert MH. Levator transposition and frontalis sling procedure in severe unilateral ptosis and the paradoxically innervated levator. *Arch Ophthalmol* 1982; **100**:462–4.

Fasanella RM, Servat J. Levator resection for minimal ptosis, another simplified procedure. *Arch Ophthalmol* 1961; **65**:493–6.

Fox SA. Congenital ptosis II. Frontalis sling. *J Pediatr Ophthalmol* 1966; **3**:25–8.

Frueh BR. The mechanistic classification of ptosis. *Ophthalmology* 1980; **87**:1019–21.

Jones LT, Quickert MH, Wobig JL. The cure of ptosis by aponeurotic repair. *Arch Ophthalmol* 1975; **93**:629–34.

LeMagne J-M. Transposition of the levator muscle and its reinnervation. *Eye* 1988; **2**:189–92.

Liu D. Ptosis repair by single suture aponeurosis tuck. Surgical technique and long-term results. *Ophthalmology* 1993; **100**:251–9.

McCord CD. *Eyelid surgery: Principles and techniques.* Philadelphia: Lippincott-Raven, 1995.

Neuhaus RW. Eyelid suspension with a transposed levator palpebrae superioris muscle. *Am J Ophthalmol* 1985; **100**:308–11.

Putterman AM, Urist MJ. Müller muscle conjunctival resection. *Arch Ophthalmol* 1975; **93**:619.

Sutula FC. Histological changes in congenital and acquired blepharoptosis. *Eye* 1988; **2**:179–84.

Wilson ME, Johnson RW. Congenital Ptosis. Long-term results of treatment using lyophilised fascia lata for frontalis suspensions. *Ophthalmology* 1991; **98**:1234–7.

6 Tumour management and repair after tumour excision

Brian Leatherbarrow

Eyelid tumours can be benign or malignant. It is not always easy clinically to differentiate between them. The consequence of failure to identify a malignant tumour in its early stages can be severe.

Malignant tumours

The appropriate management of malignant eyelid tumours requires an understanding of their clinical and pathologic characteristics. Malignant tumours affecting the eyelids are generally slowly enlarging, destructive lesions that distort or frankly destroy eyelid anatomy. Subtle features can help to differentiate malignant from benign eyelid tumours (Box 6.1). Early diagnosis can significantly reduce morbidity and indeed mortality associated with malignant eyelid tumours. However, malignant eyelid tumours are diagnosed early only if a high degree of clinical suspicion is applied to all eyelid lesions.

Slit lamp examination can highlight these various features that help to differentiate benign from malignant tumours (Figure 6.1).

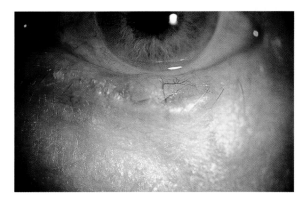

Figure 6.1 Eyelid BCC showing the malignant features of loss of lashes, obliteration of eyelid margin and pearly telangiectatic change.

Box 6.1 Clinical signs suggestive of malignancy

- A localised loss of lashes
- Obliteration of the eyelid margin
- Pearly telangiectatic change
- A new enlarging pigmented lesion
- An area of diffuse induration
- A scirrhous retracted area

Box 6.2 Malignant eyelid tumours

Epithelial
- Basal cell carcinoma
- Squamous cell carcinoma
- Sebaceous gland carcinoma

Non-epithelial
- Lymphoma – mycosis fungoides
- Merkel cell tumour
- Kaposi sarcoma
- Metastatic tumours
- Malignant sweat gland tumours
- Melanoma

Benign tumours

Most benign eyelid tumours can be readily diagnosed on the basis of their typical clinical appearance and behaviour. A number of lesions, however, cannot be easily and reliably differentiated from malignant eyelid lesion and require a biopsy for example, a keratoacanthoma. For small lesions an *excisional* biopsy serves two functions: diagnosis and treatment. For larger lesions an *incisional* biopsy is undertaken for diagnostic purposes. Conversely, some malignant lesions may appear relatively innocuous.

It is important that biopsies are performed meticulously or errors in diagnosis will occur. The tissue must be handled very carefully in order not to induce crush artefact. The tissue sample should be of adequate size and depth and ideally should include adjacent normal eyelid tissue. This is of particular importance with regard to biopsies of suspect keratoacanthoma. If a sebaceous gland carcinoma is suspected it is important to alert the pathologist of this suspicion so that appropriate stains are utilised. Some biopsy material may need to be presented on filter paper because of the very small size of the samples for example, random conjunctival sac biopsies in cases of suspected diffuse sebaceous gland carcinoma. It is important to orientate tissue for the pathologist where biopsies are attempted excisional biopsies, in case one or more edges are not clear of tumour involvement. Sutures of various lengths can be employed as markers for this purpose. A tumour excision map should be enclosed with the pathology form to assist the pathologist.

Benign tumours of the eyelids may be derived from the epidermis, dermis, adnexa (sweat glands, hair follicles, sebaceous glands), or pigment cells. There are a large number of such tumours. A few examples are shown in Box 6.3.

Basal cell carcinoma (BCC)

BCCs account for approximately 90% of malignant eyelid tumours. Ultraviolet light

---

Box 6.3 Benign eyelid tumours

A Benign lesions of the epidermis
- Achrocordon (skin tag)
- Seborrheic keratosis
- Keratoacanthoma
- Inverted follicular keratosis
- Cutaneous horn

B Benign lesions of the dermis
- Dermatofibroma
- Neurofibroma
- Capillary hemangioma
- Pyogenic granuloma
- Xanthelasma
- Xanthoma
- Juvenile xanthogranuloma

C Benign lesions of the adnexa
    Tumours of sweat gland origin
- Syringoma
- Eccrine spiradenoma

    Tumours of hair follicle origin
- Trichofolliculoma
- Pilomatrixoma

    Tumours of sebaceous gland origin
- Sebaceous gland hyperplasia
- Sebaceous adenoma

D Benign pigmentary lesions
- Nevocellular nevi
    Junction nevus
    Compound nevus
    Intradermal nevus
- Congenital nevus
- Blue nevus
- Lentigo simplex
- Lentigo senilis

---

exposure is an important aetiologic factor in the development of eyelid epithelial malignancies. This tumour is prevalent in fair-skinned people. The effects of sun exposure are cumulative, as reflected in the increasing incidence of the tumour with advancing age. BCC may, however, occur in younger patients, particularly those with a tumour diathesis such as the basal cell carcinoma syndrome.

In descending order of frequency, BCCs involve the following locations (Figure 6.2):

- Lower eyelid
- Medial canthus
- Lateral canthus
- Upper eyelid.

BCCs have a variety of clinical appearances reflecting the various histopathologic patterns of the tumour. The most common presentation is a nodular pattern. The epithelial proliferation produces a solid pearly lesion contiguous with the surface epithelium. The superficial nature of telangiectatic vessels may predispose these lesions to spontaneous bleeding. With prolonged growth, central umbilication and ulceration will occur. The typical presentation is of a chronic, indurated, non-tender, raised, pearly, telangiectatic, well circumscribed lesion with an elevated surround and depressed crater-like centre (Figure 6.3).

Clinical varieties of BCCs

- Nodular
- Ulcerative
- Cystic
- Morphoeiform
- Pigmented.

The most commonly encountered morphologic patterns of basal cell carcinoma are the nodular and ulcerative forms. Nodular basal cell carcinomas may assume various clinical presentations such as papilloma (secondary to increased keratin production), a naevus (secondary to pigmentation), and a cyst (due to central tumour necrosis). The variety of clinical presentations of basal cell carcinoma accounts for the high incidence of misdiagnosis. Clinical awareness of the

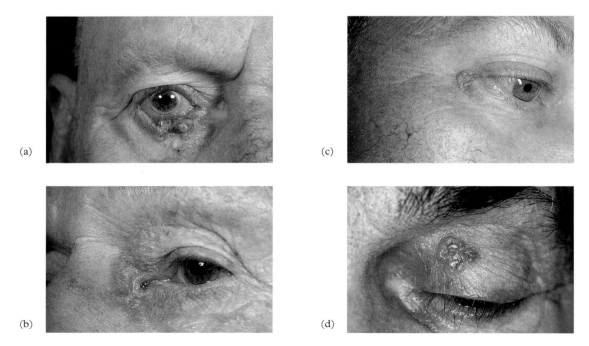

(a) (b) (c) (d)

Figure 6.2 Incidence of eyelid BCC (a) most common to (d) least common.

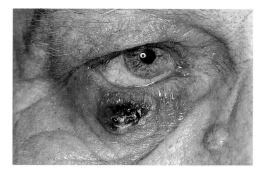

Figure 6.3   Common nodular BCC with central umbilication and ulceration.

various presentations of the tumour minimises incorrect clinical diagnoses and management.

The morphoeiform lesion has clinically indistinct margins and has a tendency to deep invasion, especially at the medial canthus. Orbital invasion by a BCC is manifest clinically as a fixed, non-mobile tumour and/or a "frozen globe". Although BCCs "never" metastasize, approximately 130 cases of metastases have been described in the literature.

The most difficult BCCs (Figure 6.4) to manage are:

- Morphoeiform BCCs
- BCCs that are fixed to bone
- Medial canthal BCCs
- BCCs with orbital invasion
- Recurrent BCCs especially following radiotherapy.

BCCs have traditionally been regarded as relatively benign, rarely invasive tumours and as such have commonly been casually excised. This has been associated with a high incidence of recurrence, unnecessary morbidity, and occasionally avoidable mortality. A dedicated approach to tumour eradication is clearly essential in the management of these patients.

Squamous cell carcinoma (SCC)

Squamous cell carcinoma in the eyelids is similar to that occurring elsewhere on the skin, with low metastatic potential and low tumour-induced mortality. It represents approximately 1–2% of all malignant eyelid lesions. The tumours tend to spread to

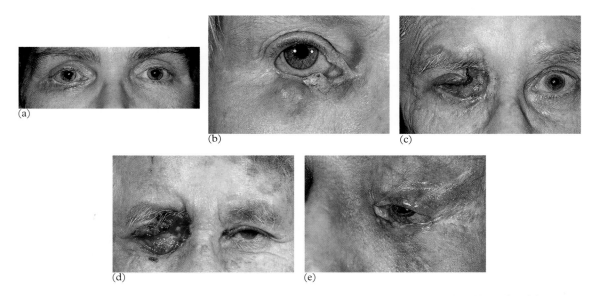

Figure 6.4   Complex BCCs, (a) morphoeic (b) fixed to bone (c) medial canthal (d) orbital invasion (e) recurrent after irradiation.

regional nodes but direct perineural invasion into the CNS is usually the cause of death in this group of patients. The tumour occurs with increasing frequency with advancing age. Radiation therapy is a significant aetiologic factor in the production of squamous cell carcinoma.

There is no pathognomonic presentation. These tumours tend to appear as thick, erythematous, elevated lesions with indurated borders and with a scaly surface (Figure 6.5). Cutaneous horn formation or extensive keratinisation are the most consistent features. When it occurs at the eyelid margin the lashes are destroyed. Squamous cell carcinomas may be derived from actinic keratoses. With chronicity and cicatricial changes of the skin, secondary ectropion may occur. The clinical features of the tumour are an exaggeration of those found with actinic keratosis.

Benign tumours such as keratoacanthoma, inverted follicular keratosis, and pseudo epitheliomatous hyperplasia simulate features of squamous cell carcinoma. The common variable with these tumours is inflammation that stimulates epithelial proliferation. Clinically, rapid growth is characteristic of these benign lesions.

Sebaceous gland carcinoma (SGC)

SGCs are very rare, with a predilection for the periocular area. In addition, SGC of the eyelids has a tendency to produce widespread metastes whereas such tumours occurring elsewhere on the skin rarely metastasize. SGC occurs with increasing frequency with advancing age. The tumour has a predilection for the upper eyelid, but diffuse upper and lower eyelid involvement may occur in patients presenting with chronic blepharoconjunctivitis.

This tumour is well recognised for its ability to masquerade as chronic blepharo-conjunctivitis or recurrent chalazion (masquerade syndrome). Recurrent chalazion or atypical solid chalazions should alert the ophthalmologist to the possibility of underlying sebaceous gland carcinoma (Figure 6.6). Histopathologic features of sebaceous gland carcinoma are characteristic and may be confirmed by lipid stains (oil red O) on fresh tissue specimens. Multicentric origin is a feature of some SGCs. Clinical presentation of chronic

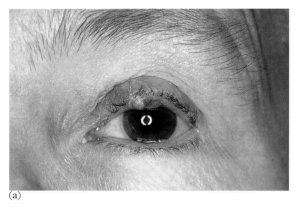

(a)

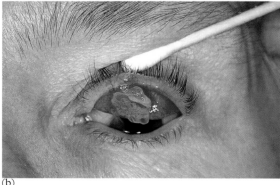

(b)

Figure 6.6 Sebaceous gland carcinoma: (a) external appearance, (b) following lid eversion.

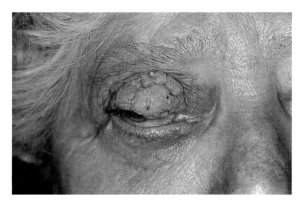

Figure 6.5 Squamous cell carcinoma.

blepharoconjunctivitis has been correlated with the pathologic features of Pagetoid involvement of the surface epithelium.

Despite the characteristic features, the tumour is frequently misdiagnosed. The aggressive behaviour and significant morbidity and mortality associated with SGCs have traditionally been attributed to the misdiagnosed tumours. The 5 year survival is 30–40%. It is clear that early diagnosis and appropriate therapy significantly reduce the long-term morbidity associated with this tumour.

Clinical features include

- Affects females more commonly than males
- More common in orientals
- Tends to occur in older patients
- Has a predilection for the upper eyelid
- Arises most commonly from the meibomian glands
- Has a lesser tendency to ulcerate
- Masquerades as recurrent chalazion or chronic blepharoconjunctivitis (Masquerade syndrome)
- May metastasize prior to establishing correct diagnosis
- High incidence of metastases
- Difficult delineation of tumour margins due to intraeithelial Pagetoid spread and/or multicentric pattern
- May be misdiagnosed histologically especially if lipid stains are not used on properly prepared tissue.

Poor prognostic factors include

- Invasion – vascular, lymphatic, or orbital
- Diffuse involvement of both eyelids
- Multicentric origin
- Tumour diameter > 10mm
- Symptoms present > 6 months

Note:

- In the Pagetoid pattern there is often involvement of both eyelids as well as the conjunctiva.

- Approximately 30% of sebaceous gland carcinomas recur.
- Systemic extension occurs by contiguous growth, lymphatic spread, and haematogenous seeding.
- The tumour spreads mainly to the orbit, the preauricular/submandibular nodes or parotid gland – less frequently to the cervical nodes, lung, pleura, liver, brain and skull.
- Some patients remain alive and well for long periods with regional node involvement – radical neck dissection for isolated cervical node disease is often indicated.
- Mortality is approximately 20–30% mainly due to late diagnosis.

Diagnosis:
A high index of suspicion is required.

- Shave biopsy – may only show inflammation
- Full thickness eyelid biopsy is required
- Random conjunctival biopsies
- Fat stains – *alert the pathologist*

Melanoma

Melanomas represent less than 1% of malignant eyelid tumours (Figure 6.7). Pigmented BCCs are ten times more common than melanoma as a cause of pigmented eyelid tumours. Forty per cent of eyelid melanomas are, however, non-pigmented.

Clinical features

- Irregular borders
- Variegated pigmentation often with inflammation
- Occasional bleeding
- Ulceration.

Occasionally the eyelid may be secondarily involved by a conjunctival melanoma.

Classification:

- Lentigo maligna melanoma
- Superficial spreading melanoma
- Nodular melanoma.

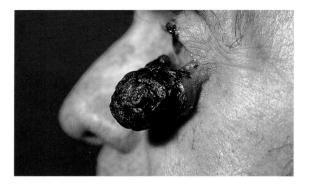

Figure 6.7   Nodular malignant melanoma.

Superficial spreading melanoma appears typically as a brown lesion with shades of red, white and blue – it is initially flat but becomes nodular with increase in vertical growth. Nodular melanoma appears as a nodule or plaque, is dark brown or black in colour but can be amelanotic. It shows little radial growth, but extensive vertical growth (Figure 6.7).

Two classic histologic classifications are based on:

- Anatomic level of involvement (Clark)
- Tumour thickness (Breslow).

Tumour thickness is the most important predictor of prognosis. The average time to metastasis for cutaneous melanomas varies according to tumour thickness. The late onset of widespread disease is rare (cf. choroidal melanomas).

Metastatic eyelid tumours

Metastatic eyelid tumours are very rare. Bronchus and breast account for 80%. The majority of patients have other known metastases at the time of presentation. The average patient survival is less than one year.

Clinical features

There is no pathognomonic presentation. A nodular/diffuse induration which may mimic a chalazion is usual.

Kaposi's sarcoma

This tumour was first described in 1872. Prior to 1981 most cases occurred in elderly Italian/Jewish men or African children. It very rarely involved periocular structures prior to AIDS but is now a relatively common manifestation of AIDS.

Clinical features

Lesions tend to be violaceous in colour (Figure 6.8). The conjunctiva may be diffusely involved and simulate inflammation.

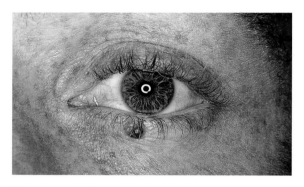

Figure 6.8   Violaceous Kaposi's sarcoma.

Rare eyelid malignancies

- Merkel cell tumour
- Lymphoid tumours – mycosis fungoides.

Such rare eyelid tumours are usually only diagnosed on histologic examination and do not tend to have pathognomonic clinical features. The Merkel cell tumour is highly malignant in its behaviour (Figure 6.9).

Principles of management for malignant eyelid tumours

The management of all malignant eyelid tumours depends on:

- Correct histological diagnosis
- Assessment of tumour margins
- Assessment of systemic tumour spread

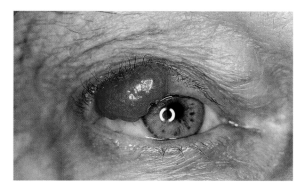

Figure 6.9   Red Merkel cell tumour.

Focal malignancy can be treated with:

- Surgery
- Radiation
- Cryotherapy.

The choice of therapy depends on:

- The size of the tumour
- The location of the tumour
- The type of tumour
- The age and general health of the patient
- The clinician's relative expertise.

The choice of treatment is particularly important in:

- Diffuse tumours
- Tumour extension to bone/the orbit
- Patients with a cancer diathesis for example, the basal cell nevus syndrome.

A comprehensive examination of the patient is important with palpation of the regional lymph nodes and a whole body skin examination wherever possible. If orbital invasion is suspected from clinical examination, for example restriction of ocular motility, it is appropriate to request thin section, high resolution CT scans with bone windows. In selected cases chest and abdominal CT is required plus liver function tests to evaluate systemic spread. If systemic spread is found, palliation only may be preferable.

Basal cell carcinoma

Management:

- Surgery in conjunction with histologic monitoring of tumour margins
- Radiation
- Cryotherapy.

The surgical management of basal cell carcinoma consists of surgical removal of the tumour with monitoring of the excised margins, either by permanent or frozen section. In the majority of cases the diagnosis is evident on clinical grounds alone. Where the diagnosis is unclear, a biopsy should be performed before definitive treatment. Although Mohs micrographic surgery is now considered by many to represent the *gold standard* in the management of periocular basal cell carcinomas, this treatment modality is unavailable in many centres in this and other countries.

Although it is reasonable to close small defects immediately, no defect should be formally reconstructed without definitive histopathological evidence of complete tumour clearance. Exenteration is reserved for cases where orbital invasion has occurred and aggressive surgical management is appropriate for the individual patient.

Tumours which recur after radiation are often poorly controlled with other modalities.

Squamous cell carcinoma

Management:

- Surgery in conjunction with histologic monitoring of tumour margins
- Irradiation.

The surgical management of squamous cell carcinoma consists of surgical removal of the tumour with monitoring of the excised margins, either by permanent or frozen section. If a biopsy of a suspicious tumour is done before a definitive surgical procedure, care should be taken to obtain a representative section of the tumour. Shave biopsies do not allow determination of dermal invasion by the epithelial tumour. Benign tumours such as actinic keratosis, kerato-acanthoma, inverted follicular keratosis, and pseudo-epitheliomatous hyperplasia can be differentiated only by evaluation of dermal extension. As such, the pathologist is frequently forced to give a diagnosis of squamous carcinoma because inadequate tissue has been submitted for review. It is not unusual for a tumour that has been reported as squamous cell carcinoma to have resolved by the time definitive surgical resection can be scheduled, for this reason.

If the lesion is small an excisional biopsy with direct closure of the defect should be performed. If the lesion is larger, an incisional biopsy should be performed. The specimen should be handled with care to avoid any crush artefact. If the lesion involves the eyelid margin, the biopsy should be full-thickness. Wherever possible, the base of the lesion and adjacent normal tissue should be included. "Laissez-faire" is useful for healing of many biopsy sites.

As in the management of BCC, Mohs' surgery is the *gold standard*. Exenteration is reserved for cases where orbital invasion has occurred and aggressive surgical management is appropriate for the individual patient.

Sebaceous gland carcinoma

Management:

- Surgery
- Irradiation.

It is important to routinely examine for evidence of pagetoid spread/multicentric origin by performing random conjunctival sac biopsies. It is appropriate to biopsy any areas of telangiectasia, papillary change or mass.

The management of SGC consists of surgical extirpation of the tumour. With heightened appreciation of the clinical presentation of the tumour, early surgical excision significantly enhances the long-term prognosis. Numerous procedures for incision and drainage of suspected recurrent chalazia delay the appropriate diagnosis of sebaceous gland carcinoma.

Localised sebaceous gland carcinoma is managed by a biopsy to establish the diagnosis with excision and monitoring of the surgical margins. A full-thickness block resection of the eyelid is usually required to establish the diagnosis. Because of the occasional multicentric presentation of sebaceous gland carcinoma, it is important to perform random conjunctival sac biopsies which should be carefully mapped and recorded. Close post operative observation is always crucial in the management of these patients to exclude recurrent disease. In patients with diffuse eyelid/conjunctival involvement or orbital extension, orbital exenteration is recommended.

Radiation therapy has a limited role in the management of SGC. The tumour is radio-sensitive and does respond to radiation therapy, but recurrences are inevitable. In addition, patients have significant ocular complications such as keratitis, radiation retinopathy, and severe pain. Radiation therapy is therefore considered a palliative procedure to reduce tumour size. It should not be viewed as a curative modality.

Melanoma

Management:

- Surgery.

The extent of tumour free margins does not correlate with survival. It is therefore appropriate to take relatively small tissue margins to preserve eyelid function wherever possible. If the tumour has extended to Clark level IV or V or its thickness exceeds 1·5mm a referral for lymph node dissection should be considered.

Radiotherapy is rarely used in the management of eyelid melanoma. Doses sufficient to destroy the tumour will destroy the eye/ocular adnexae.

Metastatic eyelid tumours

The management of metastatic eyelid tumours is the realm of the oncologist and usually involves chemotherapy and/or radiation therapy. Surgical excision can be considered if the tumour is localised and unresponsive to other modalities.

Lymphoma

The management of eyelid lymphoma is also the realm of the oncologist.

Kaposi's sarcoma

Local control is usually easily achieved with radiation.

Specific therapies

Radiation

Historically, irradiation enjoyed significant popularity among a large segment of the medical community for the treatment of epithelial malignancies, and a number of studies reported better than 90% cure rates for periocular basal cell carcinomas. More recently, however, investigators have observed that basal cell carcinomas treated by irradiation recur at a higher rate and behave more aggressively than tumours treated by surgical excision.

The radiation dose used to treat patients varies depending on the size of the lesion and the estimate of its depth. The treatments are usually fractionated over several weeks. The proponents of radiation therapy point to the lack of discomfort with radiation treatment and to the fact that no hospitalisation or anaesthesia is required.

Although radiation therapy is not recommended as the treatment of choice for periocular cutaneous malignancies, there are occasionally patients who, for various reasons, cannot undergo surgical excision and reconstruction and for whom radiation may be useful. However, it is important to continue to look closely for evidence of recurrence well beyond the five-year post operative period routinely utilised for surgically managed cutaneous malignancies.

It is now generally accepted that basal cell carcinomas recurring after radiation therapy are more difficult to diagnose, present at a more advanced stage, cause more extensive destruction, and are much more difficult to eradicate. The greater extent of destruction may be explained by the presence of adjacent radiodermatitis, which may mask underlying tumour recurrence and allow the tumour to grow more extensively before it can be clinically detected (Figure 6.10). The damaging effect of radiation on periocular tissues poses another drawback to its use.

Note the potential complications associated with the use of irradiation for treatment of periocular malignancy (Box 6.4).

The most serious complications occur after treatment of large tumours of the upper eyelid even when the eye is shielded.

Although most surgeons would oppose the use of radiotherapy as the primary modality in treating periocular skin cancers, it is felt to be

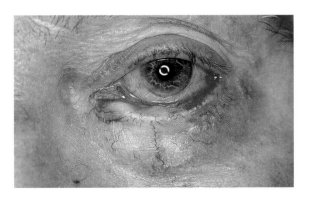

Figure 6.10   Recurrent BCC post irradiation.

Box 6.4 Potential complications of eyelid irradiation

- Skin necrosis
- Cicatricial ectropion
- Telangiectasia
- Epiphora
- Loss of lashes
- Keratitis
- Cataract
- Dry eye
- Keratinisation of the palpebral conjunctiva.

---

specifically contraindicated for lesions in the medial canthus, lesions greater than 1 cm and recurrent tumours.

Although a number of studies reported high success rates with radiation for periocular basal cell carcinomas, many of these studies did not include long-term follow-up. Investigators have now determined that it may take longer for a recurrence of a radiation-treated malignancy to become clinically apparent than for a surgically treated tumour. Recent studies with longer follow-up have reported a recurrence rate between 17% and 20%.

The radiation changes induced in surrounding tissue make it more difficult to track recurrent tumours micrographically and render subsequent reconstruction after excision more difficult. It has also been reported that radiation therapy may disturb the protective barrier offered by the periosteum and allow for greater likelihood of bony cancerous involvement with recurrences. A final concern with radiation therapy, which is not shared by other treatment modalities, is the fact that the treatment itself may induce new tumour formation.

Cryotherapy

Cryotherapy is an effective alternative therapy for small localised BCCs, especially those located in the vicinity of the puncta/canaliculi which are relatively resistant to damage by the temperatures required to kill tumour cells. It is useful in debilitated patients who are unfit for surgery. It is a single session treatment (cf. radiotherapy). A diagnostic biopsy should be performed prior to treatment. The entire tumour must be frozen to $-30°C$. Liquid nitrogen is the most effective freezing agent. The globe and adjacent tissue must be adequately protected. A thermocouple should be used and a cycle of freeze/thaw, freeze/thaw utilised.

There is an approximate 10% recurrence rate due to the inadvertent inclusion of morpheaform/diffuse tumours. There is a profound tissue reaction to cryotherapy with exudation and a prolonged period of healing.

Note the potential complications associated with the use of cryotherapy for treatment of periocular malignancy.

Box 6.5 Potential complications of cryotherapy

- Eyelid notching
- Ectropion
- Hypertrophic scarring
- Pseudoepitheliomatous hyperplasia
- Symblephara

Pseudoepitheliomatous hyperplasia is difficult to manage as it can mimic recurrent tumour.

Mohs' micrographic surgery

Mohs' micrographic surgery is a refinement of frozen-section control of tumour margins that, by mapping tumour planes, allows a three-dimensional assessment of tumour margins rather than the two-dimensional analysis provided by routine frozen section. In this technique, the surgical removal of the tumour is performed by a dermatological surgeon with specialised training in tumour excision and mapping of margins.

The unique feature of Mohs' micrographic surgery is that it removes the skin cancer in a sequence of horizontal layers, monitored by microscopic examination of horizontal sections through the undersurface of each layer. Careful mapping of residual cancer in each layer is possible, and subsequent horizontal layers are then excised in cancer-bearing areas until cancer-free histologic layers are obtained at the base and on all sides of the skin cancer.

Mohs' micrographic excision has been shown to give the highest cure rate for most cutaneous malignancies occurring on various body surfaces. In addition to its high cure rate, the technique offers several other advantages. The Mohs' technique obviates the need to remove generous margins of clinically normal adjacent tissue by allowing precise layer-by-layer mapping of tumour cells. This is extremely important in the periocular regions because of the specialised nature of the periocular tissues and the challenges in creating ready substitutes that will obtain a satisfactory functional and cosmetic result.

Because routine frozen-section monitoring of periocular skin cancers in the operating theatre involves a significant loss of time while waiting for turnaround of results from the pathologist, Mohs' micrographic excision performed in the dermatologist's minor operating theatre allows for more efficient use of operating theatre time.

Although small lesions may be allowed to granulate, excision in the majority of periocular cases is followed by immediate or next day reconstruction, by a separate oculoplastic surgeon who has expertise in reconstructing periocular defects. Reconstruction can be scheduled immediately following Mohs' micrographic excision or on a subsequent day with better prediction of the operating theatre time required. Taking responsibility for tumour excision out of the hands of the reconstructing surgeon also ensures that concerns over the difficulties of reconstruction do not limit aggressive tissue removal where it is required.

Mohs' micrographic excision has been shown to provide the most effective treatment for non-melanoma cutaneous malignancies i.e. basal cell and squamous cell carcinomas. It is not suitable for the management of sebaceous gland carcinomas. However, it is particularly recommended for the following types of periocular cutaneous malignancy:

- Skin tumours arising in the medial canthal region, where, because of natural tissue planes, the risk of deeper invasion is greater and where the borders of involved tissue are more difficult to define
- Recurrent skin tumours
- Large primary skin tumours of long duration
- Morphoeiform basal cell carcinomas
- Any tumours whose clinical borders are not obviously demarcated
- Tumours in young patients.

Although Mohs' micrographic surgery allows for the most precise histologic monitoring, some cancer cells may rarely be left behind and a 2% to 3% long-term recurrence rate has been reported for primary periocular skin cancers. Careful follow-up, searching for early signs of recurrence, remains important. One criticism of Mohs' micrographic surgery is that the surgical excision and surgical reconstruction are usually divided between two surgeons and often at two different physical sites. Some surgeons and patients find this inconvenient. In addition, Mohs' micrographic surgeons are not available in many centres in the UK and other countries.

Eyelid reconstruction

The goals in eyelid reconstruction following eyelid tumour excision are preservation of normal eyelid function for the protection of the eye and restoration of good cosmesis. Of these goals preservation of normal function is of the utmost importance and takes priority over the cosmetic result. Failure to maintain normal eyelid function, particularly following upper eyelid reconstruction, will have dire consequences for the comfort and visual performance of the patient. In general it is technically easier to reconstruct eyelid defects following tumour excision surgery than following trauma.

General principles

There are a number of surgical procedures, which can be utilised to reconstruct eyelid defects. In general, where less than 25% of the eyelid has been sacrificed, direct closure of the eyelid is possible. Where the eyelid tissues are very lax, direct closure may be possible for much larger defects occupying up to 50% of the eyelid. Where direct closure without undue tension on the wound is difficult, a simple lateral canthotomy and cantholysis of the appropriate limb of the lateral canthal tendon can effect a simple closure.

In order to reconstruct eyelid defects involving greater degrees of tissue loss, a number of different surgical procedures have been devised. The choice depends on:

- The extent of the eyelid defect
- The state of the remaining periocular tissues
- The visual status of the fellow eye
- The age and general health of the patient
- The surgeon's own expertise.

In deciding which procedure is most suited to the individual patient's needs, one should aim to re-establish the following:

- A smooth mucosal surface to line the eyelid and protect the cornea
- An outer layer of skin and muscle
- Structural support between the two lamellae of skin and mucosa originally provided by the tarsal plate

- A smooth, nonabrasive eyelid margin free from keratin and trichiasis
- In the upper eyelid normal vertical eyelid movement without significant ptosis or lagophthalmos
- Normal horizontal tension with normal medial and lateral canthal tendon positions
- Normal apposition of the eyelid to the globe
- A normal contour to the eyelid.

Large eyelid defects generally require composite reconstruction in layers with a variety of tissues, either from adjacent sources or from distant sites, being used to replace both the anterior and posterior lamellae. It is essential that only one lamella should be reconstructed as a free graft. The other lamella should be reconstructed as a vascularised flap to provide an adequate blood supply to prevent necrosis.

Lower eyelid reconstruction

Defects of the lower eyelid can be divided into those that involve the eyelid margin, and those that do not.

Defects involving the eyelid margin

a) Small defects

An eyelid defect of 25% or less may be closed directly. In patients with marked eyelid laxity, even a defect occupying up to 50% of the eyelid may be closed directly. The two edges of the defect should be grasped and pulled together to judge the facility of closure. If there is no excess tension on the lid, the edges may be approximated directly. The lid margin is reapproximated with a single armed 5/0 Vicryl suture on a half circle needle. This is passed through the most superior aspect of the tarsus, ensuring that the suture is anterior to the conjunctiva to avoid contact with the cornea. This suture is tied with a single throw and the eyelid margin approximation checked. If this is unsatisfactory the suture is replaced and the process repeated.

Once the margin approximation is good, the suture is untied and the ends fixated to the head drape with a haemostat. This elongates the wound enabling further single armed Vicryl sutures to be placed in the lower tarsus. These are tied. The uppermost Vicryl suture is then tied. Improper placement or tying of the suture or too great a degree of tension on the wound will result in dehiscence of the wound. Next, a 6/0 silk suture is passed in a vertical mattress fashion along the lash line and a second suture along the line of the meibomian glands. These are tied with sufficient tension to cause eversion of the edges of the eyelid margin wound. A small amount of pucker is desirable initially, to avoid late lid notching as the lid heals and the wound contracts. The sutures are left long and incorporated into the skin closure sutures to prevent contact with the cornea. The conjunctiva is left to heal spontaneously without suture closure. The skin sutures may be removed in five to seven days but the eyelid margin sutures should be left in place for 14 days.

b) Moderate defects

Canthotomy and cantholysis – where an eyelid defect cannot be closed directly without undue tension on the wound, a lateral canthotomy and inferior cantholysis (Figures 6.11 and 6.12) can be performed. The inferior cantholysis is performed by cutting the tissue between the conjunctiva and the skin close to the periosteum of the lateral orbital margin, with the lateral lid margin drawn up and medially.

A *semicircular flap* (Tenzel flap) (Figure 6.13) is useful for the reconstruction of defects up to 70% of the lower eyelid where some tarsus remains on either side of the defect, particularly where the patient's fellow eye has poor vision. Under these circumstances it is preferable to avoid a procedure which necessitates closure of the eye for a period of some weeks. A semicircular incision is made starting at the lateral canthus, curving superiorly to a level just below the brow and temporally for approximately 2cm.

The flap is widely undermined to the depth of the superficial temporalis fascia taking care not to damage the temporal branch of the facial nerve which crosses the midportion of the zygomatic arch. A lateral canthotomy and inferior cantholysis are then performed. The eyelid defect is closed as described above. The lateral canthus is suspended with a deep 5/0 Vicryl suture passed through the upper limb of the lateral canthal tendon or the periosteum of the lateral orbital margin to prevent retraction of the flap. Any residual dog ear is removed and the lateral skin wound closed with simple interrupted sutures.

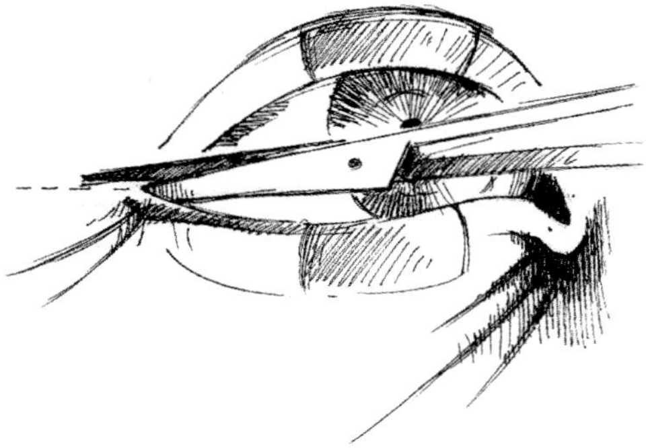

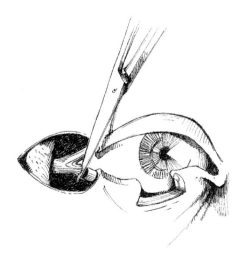

Figure 6.11   Lateral canthotomy.

Figure 6.12   Inferior cantholysis.

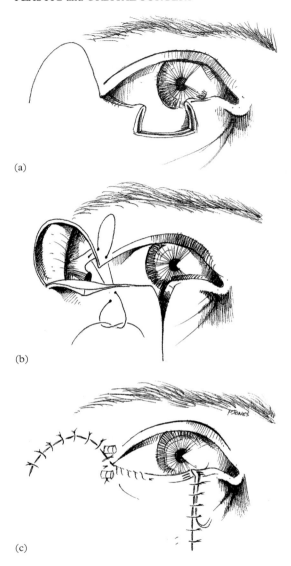

(a)

(b)

(c)

Figure 6.13 Semicircular flap for reconstruction of defects of the lower eyelid: (a) semicircular flap delineated, (b) reformation of lateral canthus, (c) sutured flap.

c) Large defects

The *upper lid tarsoconjunctival pedicle flap* (Hughes' flap) (Figure 6.14) is an excellent technique for the reconstruction of relatively shallow defects involving up to 100% of the eyelid. With defects extending horizontally beyond the eyelids it can be combined with periosteal flaps from the canthi to recreate

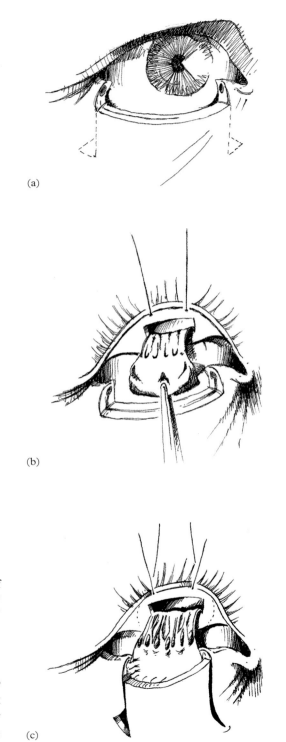

(a)

(b)

(c)

Figure 6.14 Hughes' flap: (a) following excision of lid lesion, (b) tarsoconjunctival flap raised from upper lid, and (c) sutured to posterior lamella of lower lid.

canthal tendons. *Great care, however, should be taken in the planning and construction of the flap in order not to compromise the function of the upper eyelid.*

A 4/0 silk traction suture is passed through the grey line of the upper eyelid which is everted over a Desmarres retractor. The size of the flap to be constructed is ascertained by pulling together the edges of the eyelid wound firmly and measuring the residual defect. A horizontal incision is made centrally through the tarsus 3·5mm above the lid margin. It is important to leave a tarsal height of 3·5mm below the incision in order to prevent an upper eyelid entropion and to prevent any compromise of the eyelid margin blood supply. The horizontal incision is completed with blunt-tipped Westcott scissors, and vertical relieving cuts are made at both ends of the tarsal incision. The tarsus and conjunctiva are dissected free from Müller's muscle and the levator aponeurosis up to the superior fornix.

The tarsoconjunctival flap is mobilised into the lower lid defect. The tarsus is sutured to the lower lid tarsus with interrupted 5/0 Vicryl sutures. The lower lid conjunctival edge is sutured to the inferior border of the mobilised tarsus with a continuous 7/0 Vicryl suture.

Sufficient skin to cover the anterior surface of the flap can be obtained either by harvesting a full-thickness skin graft or by advancing a myocutaneous flap from the cheek (Figure 6.15). This flap can be elevated by bluntly dissecting a skin and muscle flap inferiorly, toward the orbital rim, and incising the lid and cheek skin vertically. Relaxing triangles (Burrow's triangles) may be excised on the inferior medial and lateral edges of the defect. The flap of skin and muscle is then advanced with sufficient undermining so that it will lie in place without tension. This flap is then sewn in place with its upper border at the appropriate level to produce the new lower lid margin.

In the patient with relatively tight, non-elastic skin, such an advancement may

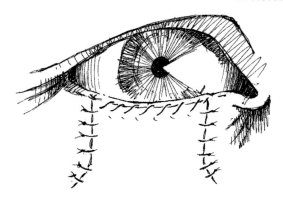

Figure 6.15 Hughes' reconstruction with skin/muscle advancement flap.

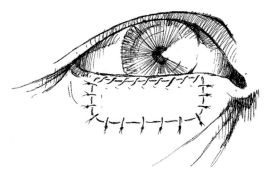

Figure 6.16 Hughes' reconstruction with full-thickness skin graft.

eventually lead to eyelid retraction or an ectropion. In such cases, it is wiser to use a free full thickness skin graft from the opposite upper lid, pre-auricular area, retro-auricular area or from the upper inner arm area (Figure 6.16). The graft should not be taken from the upper lid of the same eye as the Hughes' flap, as the resultant vertical shortening of both the anterior and the posterior lamellae may produce vertical contracture of the donor lid. If possible, a flap of orbicularis muscle can be advanced alone after dissecting it free from overlying skin. This will improve the vascular recipient bed for the skin graft. If a full-thickness skin graft has been utilised, an occlusive dressing is applied for five to seven days. Skin sutures may be removed after five to seven days. The patient is instructed to massage the area in an upward direction for a few minutes, three to four times per day to keep the tissues supple and prevent undue contracture.

The flap can be opened approximately six to eight weeks (or longer if necessary) after surgery. This is done by inserting one blade of a pair of blunt-tipped Westcott scissors just above the desired level of the new lid border and cutting the flap open. It is unnecessary to angle the scissors to leave the conjunctival edge somewhat higher than the anterior edge. Traditionally this provides some conjunctiva posteriorly to be draped forward and create a new mucocutaneous lid margin, but this leaves a reddened lid margin which is cosmetically poor. It is preferable to allow the lid margin simply to granulate as the appearance is far better. The upper lid is then everted and the residual flap is excised flush to its attachment. If Müller's muscle has been left undisturbed in the original dissection of the flap, eyelid retraction is minimal and no formal attempt is needed to recess the upper lid retractors. The Hughes' procedure provides excellent cosmetic and functional results for lower lid reconstruction.

Free tarsoconjunctival graft – adequate tarsal support may be provided by harvesting a free tarsoconjunctival graft from either upper lid. The upper lid is everted as described above. The size of the graft needed is determined in a similar manner as well. Again, the tarsus is incised across the width of the lid, 3 to 4mm above the lash line, to prevent upper lid instability and lash loss. The flap is elevated by blunt dissection in the pretarsal space, and vertical cuts are made to the tarsal base. The tarsus is then amputated at its base and grafted into the recipient lower lid, as described above. Because this graft is inherently avascular, it must be covered by a vascularized myocutaneous advancement flap.

This technique is useful in lower lid reconstruction for a monocular patient, because it does not occlude the visual axis. If the surgical defect extends to involve the canthal tendons, the free graft should be anchored to periosteal flaps.

Periosteal flap – for the repair of lateral lid defects in which the tarsus and the lateral canthal tendon have been completely excised, a periosteal flap provides excellent support for the reconstruction. The periosteum should be elevated as a rectangular strip from the outer aspect of the lateral orbital rim, at the midpupillary level, to provide upward support. The flap should be 4 to 5mm in height, and the length can be judged based on the size of the defect to be reconstructed. The hinged flap is elevated and folded medially and secured to the edge of the residual tarsus or to the inner aspect of a myocutaneous flap with 5/0 or 6/0 absorbable sutures.

Mustarde cheek rotation flap – with the development and popularity of other reconstruction techniques and with the tissue conserving advantages of Mohs' micrographic surgery, the Mustarde rotational cheek flap is more rarely utilised than in the past (Figure 6.17). It is reserved for the reconstruction of very extensive deep eyelid defects usually involving more than 75% of the eyelid.

A large myocutaneous cheek flap is dissected and used in conjunction with an adequate mucosal lining posteriorly. The posterior lamella tarsal substitute is usually a nasal septal cartilage graft or a hard palate graft. The important points in designing a cheek flap are summarised by Mustarde in the following points.

- A deep inverted triangle must be excised below the defect to allow adequate rotation.
- The side of the triangle nearest the nose should be practically vertical. Failure to observe this point will result in pulling down the advancing flap because the centre of rotation of the leading edge is too far to the lateral side.
- The outline of the flap should rise in a curve toward the tail of the eyebrow and hairline and should reach down as far as the lobule of the ear.

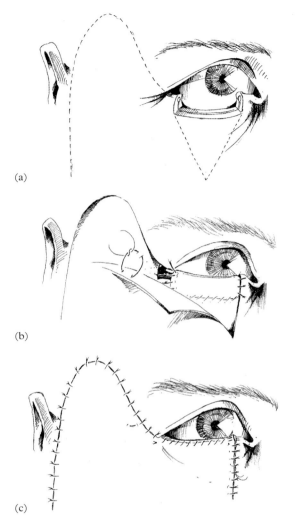

(a)

(b)

(c)

Figure 6.17 Mustarde flap: (a) delineated, (b) advanced following final reconstruction of posterior lamella, (c) skin sutures.

- The flap must be adequately undermined from the lowest point of the incision in front of the ear across the whole cheek to within 1cm below the apex of the excised triangle.
- Where necessary (in defects of three quarters or more), a back cut should be made at the lowest point, 1cm or more below the lobule of the ear.
- The deep tissue of the flap should be hitched up to the orbital rim, especially at the lateral canthus, to prevent the weight of the flap from pulling on the lid.

Cheek flaps can be followed by many complications, including *facial-nerve paralysis*, necrosis of the flap, ectropion, entropion, epiphora, sagging lower lid, and excessive facial scarring. *It is very important to plan the design of the flap and to appreciate the plane of dissection to avoid inadvertent injury to the facial nerve resulting in lagophthalmos.* Meticulous attention to haemostasis is important as is placement of a drain and a compressive dressing at the conclusion of surgery.

There are a number of alternative local periocular flaps which can be utilised for anterior lamella replacement It is important to respect a length–width ratio of approximately 4:1 where such flaps are not based on an axial blood supply to avoid necrosis. A particularly useful flap is that harvested from above the brow and based temporally It provides good vertical support but requires second stage revision. Other local flaps which are harvested from the lower lateral cheek area or the nasojugal area have the disadvantage of secondary lymphoedema which can take many months to resolve.

A flap can be used from the upper eyelid where there is sufficient redundant tissue. Occasionally the flap can be created as a bucket handle based both temporally and nasally. It is essential, however, to ensure that the creation of such flaps does not cause lagophthalmos.

Eyelid defects not involving the eyelid margin

If the lid border is spared and the tumour does not invade orbicularis or deeper tissues, a full-thickness section of lid does not have to be excised. If the lesion is small, the defect may be closed with direct approximation of the skin edges after undermining. It is important to close the wound to leave a vertical scar to avoid a post operative ectropion. In large lesions, a full-thickness skin graft may be necessary to prevent ectropion of the lower lid. If the lid is lax, this may have to be combined with a lateral tarsal strip procedure or a wedge resection in order to prevent a lower eyelid ectropion.

Upper eyelid reconstruction

Reconstruction of upper eyelid tumour defects must be performed meticulously in order to avoid ocular surface complications. There are a number of surgical procedures which can be utilised to reconstruct an upper lid defect. It is important to select the procedure which is best suited to the individual patient's needs.

Lagophthalmos following reconstruction may cause exposure keratopathy, particularly in the absence of a good Bell's phenomenon. The problem is compounded by loss of accessory lacrimal tissue. Lacrimal tissue should be preserved when dissecting in the lateral canthal, lateral levator, and lateral anterior orbital areas. Poor eyelid closure is usually due either to adhesions, wound contracture, or to a vertical skin shortage. It may also be caused by overenthusiastic dissection of lateral periocular flaps with damage to branches of the facial nerve.

When levator function is preserved following surgical defects of the eyelid, ptosis can usually be avoided or corrected. It is important to carefully identify the cut edges of the levator and to ensure that the levator is reattached to the reconstructed tarsal replacement with a suitable spacer if required.

Eyelid defects involving the eyelid margin

a) Small defects

As in the lower lid reconstruction, an eyelid defect of 25% or less may be closed directly and in patients with marked eyelid laxity, even a defect occupying up to 50% of the eyelid may be closed directly (Figure 6.18). The surgical procedure is as described above. It is important that the tarsal plate is aligned precisely and closed with 5/0 Vicryl sutures, ensuring that the bites are partial thickness to avoid the possibility of corneal abrasion. After closure of the tarsus, the eyelid margin is closed with

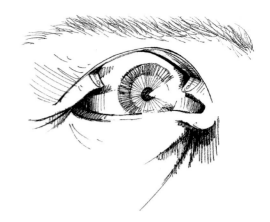

Figure 6.18   Upper eyelid defect.

interrupted 6/0 silk sutures placed at the grey line and lash margin. All eyelashes should be everted away from the cornea. The ends of the margin sutures are left long and sutured to the external skin tissue to avoid corneal irritation.

b) Moderate defects

Canthotomy and cantholysis – where an eyelid defect cannot be closed directly without undue tension on the wound, a lateral canthotomy (Figure 6.11) and superior cantholysis (Figure 6.19) can performed. It is very important that the cantholysis is performed meticulously to avoid any inadvertent damage to the levator aponeurosis or to the lacrimal gland.

Semicircular flap – a lateral, inverted, semicircular flap may be combined with direct

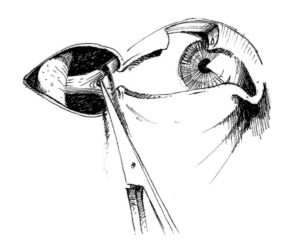

Figure 6.19   Superior cantholysis.

closure for full-thickness defects of up to two thirds of the eyelid margin (Figure 6.20a, b and c). An inverted semicircle is marked on the skin surface, beginning at the lateral canthus and extending laterally approximately 3cm. The skin and orbicularis muscle are undermined under the entire flap, and a superior cantholysis performed. The lateral aspect of the eyelid may then be advanced medially to cover the defect.

The posterior surface of the advanced semicircular flap may be covered by a tarsoconjunctival advancement flap from the lateral aspect of the lower eyelid. A vertical, full-thickness, lower eyelid incision is made, and the tarsoconjunctival advancement flap is prepared by excising the lower eyelid skin tissue and lash margin from the flap. The tarsus and conjunctiva may then be advanced superiorly into the lateral aspect of the upper eyelid flap. The lower eyelid defect may be repaired primarily, anterior to the tarsoconjunctival flap. The lateral tarsoconjunctival flap may be released in four to six weeks.

As an alternative to semicircular skin advancement, the advanced lower lid tarsoconjunctival flap may be covered with full-thickness skin tissue rather than a rotated, inverted semicircle.

c) Large defects

Sliding tarsoconjunctival flap – horizontal advancement of an upper eyelid tarsoconjunctival flap is useful for full-thickness defects of up to two thirds of the upper lid margin. The residual upper eyelid tarsus is bisected horizontally. The superior portion of the tarsus is advanced horizontally along with its levator and Müller's muscle attachments. The tarsoconjunctival advancement flap created is then sutured in a side-to-side fashion to the lower portion of the upper lid tarsus and to the lateral or medial canthal tendon. The lower portion of the upper lid tarsus remains attached to the orbicularis and skin tissue. After the horizontal tarsoconjunctival advancement, the external skin tissue is rebuilt by using full-thickness skin grafting or semicircular adjacent tissue advancement.

A *Cutler-Beard reconstruction* is useful for upper eyelid defects covering up to 100% of the eyelid margin. A three-sided inverted U-shaped incision is marked on the lower eyelid, beginning below the tarsus. The eyelid is everted over a Desmarres retractor and a conjunctival incision is made below the tarsus. A conjunctival flap is fashioned and dissected into the inferior fornix and onto the globe. The flap is advanced into the upper eyelid defect and sewn edge to edge with the remaining upper fornix conjunctiva using 7/0 Vicryl with care being taken to avoid corneal irritation (Figure 6.21a). The cornea is now protected.

Tarsal support to the upper eyelid is replaced by placing an autogenous auricular

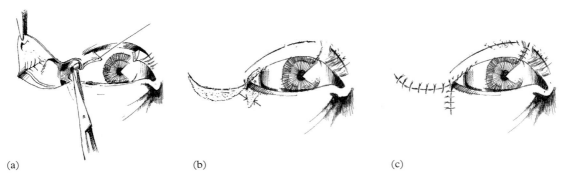

(a)   (b)   (c)

Figure 6.20   Semicircular flap reconstruction (a) with superior cantholysis, (b) with lower lid posterior lamella advancement flap, (c) final result.

cartilage graft, which has been suitably shaped, anterior to the conjunctival flap. The edges are sewn horizontally to either tarsal remnants or to periosteal flaps (Figure 6.21b). An incision is made through the lower eyelid horizontally below the tarsus and extended inferiorly to create a skin muscle advancement flap. The lower lid skin-and-muscle flap is then advanced to the upper lid to cover the cartilage graft (Figure 6.21c).

The lower lid tissue is advanced posteriorly to the remaining lower lid tarsal and lid margin bridge. The bridge flap is left intact for at least eight weeks prior to separation. When the bridge flap is separated, a full-thickness incision should be made through the flap at a position inferior to the lower lid bridge margin (Figure 6.21d). The conjunctiva and skin are then sutured directly in the newly separated upper eyelid tissue. The inferior margins of the lower lid bridge are freshened and reanastomosed to the remaining lower lid skin and conjunctival layers (Figure 6.21e). It is common for the lower lid to become very lax and to require a wedge resection at the second stage.

Full-thickness composite graft – a full-thickness en bloc section of tissue from the other upper eyelid may be transplanted into defects of the upper eyelid margin. The resection of the normal eyelid should be performed below the lid crease and should be done only when the remaining normal eyelid can be easily closed with direct closure. The lashes of the transplanted lid rarely survive. The overlying skin and orbicularis are removed and a rotation/advancement flap is fashioned to cover the graft.

Rotation and inversion of the lower lid margin and tarsus into an upper lid defect provides good lid function as well as lashes for the upper eyelid. This procedure is best used, however, for large upper lid defects. It necessitates complete reconstruction of the lower eyelid margin, utilising a lateral Mustarde cheek flap reconstruction combined with a hard palate or nasal chondromucosal graft for the reconstruction of the lower eyelid tarsus and conjunctiva. This technique is particularly useful for reconstruction of upper eyelid colobomata.

The lower lid margin needed for upper lid reconstruction is outlined laterally and a vertical full-thickness incision is made inferiorly in the lower eyelid flap. The lateral

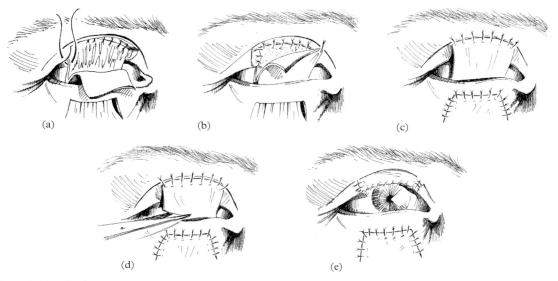

(a) (b) (c)

(d) (e)

Figure 6.21   Cutler-Beard reconstruction (a) conjunctival flap in place, (b) ear cartilage graft in place, (c) first stage complete, (d) division of Cutler-Beard flap, (e) final stage.

aspect of the lower eyelid is then advanced medially through the use of a lateral Mustarde flap. The lower eyelid margin is then inverted and sutured into the upper lid defect. The lower lid rotation is closed medially, and the lateral aspect of the new lower lid margin is backed with a nasal chondromucosal composite graft or a hard palate graft. The bridge adjoining the upper and lower lids is separated after six to eight weeks. Although some surgeons use this technique with success, it is cumbersome and requires both lower eyelid construction and lateral facial advancement.

Eyelid defects not involving the eyelid margin

If a small skin defect can be closed directly this should aim to leave a vertical scar in order to prevent vertical contracture of the wound and secondary lagophthalmos or eyelid retraction. If direct closure of the tissue is not possible, a full-thickness skin graft may be placed over the defect to prevent lagophthalmos.

Full-thickness loss of upper and lower lids

Reconstruction of the upper eyelid becomes much more of a challenge when additional periocular tissue and part of the lower eyelid have been lost. The type of reconstruction will then depend very much on the age and general health of the patient and the visual status of the fellow eye. Frequently concerns about cosmesis will have to be sacrificed to concerns about adequate corneal protection.

When a full-thickness defect includes the entire upper and lower eyelids, the goal of reconstruction becomes preservation of the globe by complete coverage with mucous membrane and skin tissue. Usually, sufficient conjunctiva is available on the bulbar surface to allow undermining and reflection over the corneal surface. The reflected bulbar conjunctiva inferiorly is sutured to the reflected conjunctiva superiorly. This can then be covered with a full-thickness skin graft or a rotation flap from the lateral face or mid-forehead. After maturation of the tissue, a small opening can be made to permit central corneal vision. Because the upper and lower eyelids are immobile, only a small palpebral fissure should be created to minimise the risk of lagophthalmos and exposure.

If available bulbar conjunctiva is insufficient to cover the globe, full-thickness buccal mucous membrane may be grafted to the posterior surface of the lateral cheek or midline forehead flap to provide a mucosal lining for the globe.

When ample conjunctiva with a good blood supply is available, the reflected mucosal covering may be adequate to support full-thickness skin grafting externally as an alternative to larger flap rotations.

Further reading

Abide JM, Nahai F, Bennett RG. The meaning of surgical margins. *Plast Reconstr Surg* 1984; **73**:492–6.

Anderson RL, Ceilley RI. Multispeciality approach to excision and reconstruction of eyelid tumours. *Ophthalmology* 1978; **85**:1150–63.

Collin JRO. *A manual of systematic eyelid surgery*. New York: Churchill Livingstone, 1989.

Cutler NL, Beard C. A method for partial and total upper lid reconstruction. *Am J Ophthalmol* 1955; **39**:1.

Gooding CA, White G, Yatsuhashi M. Significance of marginal extension in excised basal cell carcinoma. *N Engl J Med* 1965; **273**:923–5.

Hewes EH, Sullivan JH, Beard C. Lower eyelid reconstruction by tarsal transposition. *Am J Ophthalmol* 1976; **81**:512–14.

Hughes WL. *Reconstructive surery of the eyelids* (2nd ed) St. Louis: CV Mosby, 1954.

Inkster C, Ashworth J, Murdoch JR, Montgomery P, Telfer NR, Leatherbarrow B. Oculoplastic reconstruction following Mohs' surgery. *Eye* 1998; **12**:214–18.

Leshin B, Yeatts P. Management of periocular basal cell carcinoma: Mohs' micrographic surgery versus radiotherapy. I. Mohs' micrographic surgery. *Surv Ophthalmol* 1993; **38**:193–203.

Margo CE, Waltz K. Basal cell carcinoma of the eyelid and periocular skin. *Surv Ophthalmol* 1993; **38**:169–92.

Miller S. Biology of basal cell carcinoma. *J Am Acad Dermatol* 1991; **24**:1–13 (Part I), 161–75 (Part II).

Mohs FE. Micrographic surgery for the microscopically controlled excision of eyelid cancers. *Arch Ophthalmol* 1986; **104**:901–9.

Mustarde JC. *Repair and reconstruction in the orbital region*. Edinburgh: Churchill Livingstone, 1966.

Pascal RR, Hobby LW, Lattes R, Crikelair GF. Prognosis of incompletely excised versus completely excised basal cell carcinomas. *Plast Reconstr Sur* 1968; **41**:328–32.

Patrinely JR, Marines HM, Anderson RL. Skin flaps in periorbital reconstruction. *Surv Ophthalmol* 1987; **31**: 249–61.

Putterman AM. Viable composite grafting in eyelid reconstruction: a new method of upper and lower lid reconstruction. *Am J Ophthalmol* 1978; **85**:237–41.

Rakofsky SI. The adequacy of surgical excision of basal cell carcinoma. *Ann Ophthalmol* 1973; **5**:596–600.

Robins P, Rodriquez-Sains R, Rabinovitz H, Rigel D. Mohs' surgery for periocular basal cell carcinoma. *J Dermatol Surg Oncol* 1985; **11**:1203–7.

Salasche SJ, Amonette R. Morpheaform basal cell epitheliomas: A study of subclinical extensions in a series of 51 cases. *J Dermatol Surg Oncol* 1981; 7:387–92.

Tenzel RR, Stewart WB. Eyelid reconstruction by the semicircle flap technique. *Ophthalmology* 1978; **5**:1164–9.

Von Domarus H, Steven PJ. Metastatic basal cell carcinoma. Report of five cases and review of 170 cases in the literature. *J Am Acad Dermatol* 1984; **10**:1043–60.

Waltz KL Margo CE. The interpretation of microscopically controlled surgical margins (abstract). *Ophthalmology* 1991; **91**:117.

Wolf DJ, Zitelli JA. Surgical margins for basal cell carcinoma. *Arch Dermatol* 1987; **123**:340–4.

7 Seventh nerve palsy and corneal exposure

Anthony G Tyers

Seventh nerve palsy

Seventh nerve palsy is most commonly due to Bell's palsy. Less common causes include herpes zoster oticus (Ramsay-Hunt syndrome) and trauma (including surgery). Other causes, for example tumours, are less common.

The prognosis for recovery of facial function depends on the cause of the facial palsy. Bell's palsy recovers well in more than 75% of cases; however, following Ramsay-Hunt syndrome, recovery of the palsy is much less likely. In Bell's palsy the prognosis in an individual case can be estimated from the timing of the first signs of recovery: onset of recovery within three weeks – recovery is usually good; onset after six weeks – recovery is usually incomplete; no recovery by six months – the diagnosis is not Bell's palsy. Electrodiagnostic tests may also be used to estimate the prognosis.

Assessment

Patients with seventh nerve palsy may present with *a painful red eye, watering* or *cosmetic defects*. A painful red eye requires the most urgent treatment and is potentially the most dangerous; watering causes the most inconvenience, and cosmetic defects are the most difficult aspect of facial palsy to treat. An accurate history is essential. The early clinical assessment should include examination of lid function and closure, Bell's phenomenon, tear flow and corneal sensation. In Ramsay-Hunt syndrome there are usually vesicles in the external auditory meatus.

A *painful red eye* results from corneal exposure. Poor upper lid closure alone may not cause exposure but other factors precipitate it – Bell's phenomenon protects the cornea but it may be inadequate in about 10% of people; tear production is reduced in facial palsy if the lesion is proximal to the geniculate ganglion; the corneal sensation may be reduced; finally, lower lid ectropion may contribute to exposure. Reduced tear production occurs in about 15–20% of Bell's palsy patients. Corneal sensation may be reduced in Bell's palsy but it is more common in facial palsy following surgical treatment of intracranial tumours, especially acoustic neuroma.

Watering is due to loss of the lacrimal pump mechanism and it is exacerbated by lower lid ectropion. Tears are pumped from the lacus lacrimalis along the canaliculi to the lacrimal sac during blinking. Facial palsy compromises this mechanism and it may not recover even after relatively good recovery of facial function.

Watering after facial palsy may also occur if the "crocodile tear syndrome" develops. This watering is associated with eating and is believed to be due to aberrant regeneration of the parasympathetic fibres to one or more of the salivary glands which become misdirected to the lacrimal gland.

Cosmetic defects around the eyes include brow ptosis, poor upper lid function, lower lid ectropion and watering. Synkinesis, defined as an involuntary movement of part of the face other than that intended to move, can be severe and distressing, causing a significant cosmetic defect. Usually, closure of the eye also causes upward movement of the corner of the mouth, and movement of the mouth also causes closure of the eye.

Management

Treatment in the early weeks is directed at the painful red eye. Treatment for the watering and the cosmetic defects can be deferred until after six months when all likely recovery has occurred. Reassurance and support of the patient is needed at every stage.

Early management – the painful red eye

Topical lubricants and taping the eye closed at night may be all that is required. A temporary lateral tarsorrhaphy may be needed to control severe exposure while the prognosis for recovery is being assessed. Marked ectropion of the lower lid may be treated early. Simple lid shortening, as for an involutional ectropion, may be effective but a better lid position is achieved with a lateral canthal sling (Chapter 3).

Management after six months – continuing exposure; watering and cosmetic defects

Continuing exposure due to poor lid closure or an inadequate blink may be treated by lowering the upper lid, which is often slightly retracted due to the unopposed action of the levator palpebrae muscle. Müller's muscle may be recessed or excised. The upper lid may be lowered further by recession of both Müller's muscle and the levator muscle but this is rarely needed in facial palsy. Alternatively, a gold weight may be implanted into the upper lid – this allows a more natural blink and better

eyelid closure. Many other techniques have been proposed to "reanimate" the upper lid but most of these have been abandoned because of complications. The "temporalis transfer" operation is effective and is still widely used for severe exposure where expensive options such as the use of gold weights are impractical.

Ectropion is treated with a lateral canthal sling combined with a medial canthoplasty. If, however, the medial canthal tendon is very lax an alternative is a medial wedge resection. For severe and persistent ectropion the lower lid can be supported with a sling of autogenous fascia lata.

Persistent watering, if severe, is effectively treated with a Lester Jones tube.

Cosmetic improvement in seventh nerve palsy is always challenging. In addition to the procedures mentioned above, the brow position may be corrected, if necessary, with a direct brow lift. The scar heals well. However, even less scarring follows brow lifts performed through a coronal incision or an endoscopic approach which is performed through several small incisions within the hair line. These are more difficult and specialised procedures. Blepharoplasty of the lower lids may be needed if laxity in the orbicularis muscle allows bags to appear and fluid to pool in the lids. Synkinesis can be treated with botulinum toxin injections if severe.

Surgical techniques in seventh nerve palsy

Lateral tarsorrhaphy

The principle is to join the upper and lower lids laterally to reduce the palpebral aperture horizontally and improve the protection of the cornea.

The *technique* is as follows:

a) *Temporary tarsorrhaphy* (Figure 7.1a).

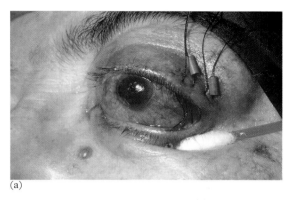

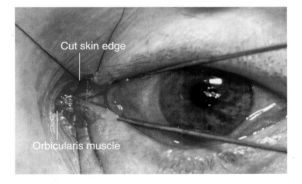

Figure 7.1 Lateral tarsorrhaphy (a) temporary, (b) permanent.

- Excise the lid margin tissues of the upper and lower lid laterally for the length of the intended tarsorrhaphy.
- Insert two vertical mattress sutures of 4/0 silk – as shown in the diagram. Tie the sutures over bolsters.
- Remove the sutures at one week.

b) *Permanent tarsorrhaphy* (Figure 7.1b).

- Make an incision along the grey line of the upper lid and lower lid laterally for the length of the intended tarsorrhaphy. Deepen the incisions, staying on the anterior tarsal surfaces for the full height of the upper and lower lid tarsal plates.
- Make a vertical cut through the full height of the upper and lower lid tarsal plates at the medial ends of the grey line incisions. This creates triangles of tarsal plate laterally in the upper and lower lids.
- Excise the triangle of the tarsal plate in the lower lid.
- Insert a double armed 4/0 suture through the tip of the triangle of the tarsal plate in the upper lid. Pass both needles through the apex of the bare area in the posterior aspect of the lower lid and through to the skin. Tie the sutures over a bolster.
- Close the skin of the lid margin with vertical mattress sutures from above the upper lid lashes to below the lower lid

lashes. This ensures the lashes do not point posteriorly to abrade the cornea.

Complications –

- Temporary tarsorrhaphy – the tarsorrhaphy often breaks down in places as soon as the sutures are removed.
- Permanent tarsorrhaphy – a fistula which drains tears may appear at the lateral canthus if the canthal skin is not carefully closed.

Medial canthoplasty (Figure 7.2)

The principle is that the margin of the upper and lower lids medial to the lacrimal puncta are joined to reduce the palpebral aperture and support the medial end of the lower lid.

Figure 7.2 Medial canthoplasty.

The *technique* is as follows:

- Place lacrimal probes in the canaliculi. Make incisions along the upper and lower lid margins medial to the puncta, staying anterior to the canaliculi, and join the incisions at the inner canthus. Undermine the skin to expose the orbicularis muscle above the below the canaliculi.
- Place one or two 6/0 absorbable sutures from the muscle above the upper canaliculus to the muscle below the lower canaliculus.
- Tie the sutures to approximate the upper and lower lids of the inner canthus.
- Close the skin with 6/0 sutures. Remove the sutures at a week.

Complications – the canthoplasty may stretch with time.

Medial wedge resection (Figure 7.3)

The principle is that stretched medial eyelid tissue, which includes the medial canthal tendon and the proximal lower lid canaliculus, is excised and the tarsal plate is reattached to the posterior lacrimal crest to create a firm support to the medial end of the lower lid.

The *technique* is as follows:

- Make a vertical cut through the full thickness of the lower lid, 4–5mm lateral to the medial canthus. Gently pull the lateral edge of the wound medially to take up the slack in the lower lid margin and excise the excess as a pentagon.
- Place a probe into the cut end of the lower canaliculus. Using blunt dissection with scissors, directed posteriorly and medially behind the canaliculus and staying lateral to the lacrimal sac, identify the posterior lacrimal crest just posterior to the sac. A narrow malleable retractor placed laterally will help visualisation of the posterior lacrimal crest.
- Insert a double armed, nonabsorbable 5/0 suture into the periostium of the posterior lacrimal crest, slightly above the level of the inner canthus.
- Pass the first needle through the tarsal plate close to the lid margin, from posterior to anterior and the second needle 2–3mm inferior to the first. Adjust the position of the two arms of the suture if necessary so that when it is tied the lid is drawn medially and posteriorly against the globe.
- Cut along the posterior wall of the cut canaliculus for 2–3mm, place a 7/0 absorbable suture between the anterior lip of the cut canaliculus and the conjunctival edge on the lower lid laterally. When this suture is tied it will turn the lumen of the canaliculus posteriorly into the conjunctival sac so that some tears will drain.
- Before tying the 5/0 suspending suture, carefully close the conjunctival wound with a 6/0 absorbable suture to ensure that the 5/0 suspending suture is well covered posteriorly. Next, tie the canalicular suture. Finally, tie the 5/0 suspending suture to fix the medial end of the lid.
- Close skin with 6/0 sutures. Remove these at one week.

Complications – the medial end of the lid may be held away from the eye if the 5/0 suspending suture is placed too far anteriorly in the posterior lacrimal crest. In addition,

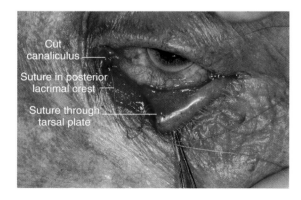

Figure 7.3   Medial wedge resection.

poor placement of the 5/0 suspending suture through the tarsal plate may cause distortion of the lid margin medially. Both of these complications can be corrected at operation by careful placement of the suture.

Inadequate closure of the conjunctiva, so that the 5/0 suture is exposed, may lead to granuloma formation. This will normally settle slowly over several weeks but may need to be excised.

Tarsotomy (Figure 7.4)

The principle is to disinsert Müller's muscle from the tarsal plate. This lowers the upper lid by up to 2mm to overcome upper lid retraction and improve closure of the eye.

The *technique* is as follows:

- Insert a traction suture through the upper lid margin. Evert the lid over a Desmarres retractor and incise the tarsal plate close to its superior border.
- Extend the incision in the tarsal plate medially and laterally, parallel to the full width of the superior tarsal border.
- Tape the traction suture firmly down to the cheek, under the dressing, for 48 to 72 hours.

Complications – the lid frequently rises to its original position once the traction suture is removed.

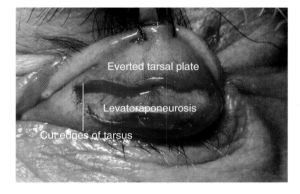

Figure 7.4   Upper lid tarsotomy.

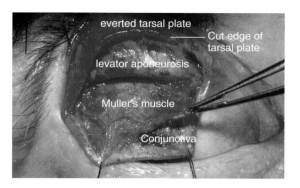

Figure 7.5   Excision of Müller's muscle.

Müller's muscle excision (Figure 7.5)

The principle is the removal of Müller's muscle to lower the lid by 2–3mm.

The *technique* is as follows:

- Follow the first two steps as for tarsotomy.
- Pull down the lower wound edge – this includes the narrow strip of the superior tarsal plate with Müller's muscle attached. Dissect in the fine connective tissue between Müller's muscle posteriorly and the levator aponeurosis anteriorly until the junction of Müller's muscle and aponeurosis is reached, after about 10mm. Carefully, dissect Müller's muscle from the conjunctiva and excise the muscle.
- Close the wound in the tarsal plate with a continuous 6/0 or 7/0 absorbable suture taking care to bury the knots at either end of the wound to avoid abrasion of the cornea.

Complications – mild persistent ptosis often follows this operation. The upper lid margin may be distorted if Müller's muscle is incompletely excised.

Gold weight implantation (Figure 7.6)

The principle is that an implanted gold weight closes the lid when the levator muscle is relaxed with blinking and voluntary eyelid closure.

71

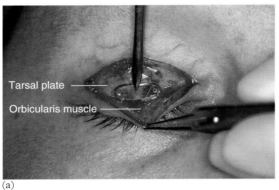

(a)

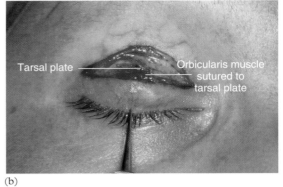

(b)

Figure 7.6   (a) Gold weight placed between the tarsal plate and orbicularis muscle, (b) orbicularis muscle sutured to tarsal plate over the gold weight.

The *technique* is as follows:

- Estimate the required weight of the implant with test weights stuck to the upper lid skin close to the lashes. The correct weight allows complete closure of the upper and lower lids but no more than a slight ptosis when the eyes are open. Order the gold implant of the correct weight.
- Make a skin crease incision, deepen it to the tarsal plate and dissect inferiorly deep to the orbicularis muscle on the surface of the tarsal plate, almost to the lid margin.
- Suture the gold weight to the tarsal plate close to the lid margin (Figure 7.6a).
- Close the orbicularis muscle of the inferior wound edge to the tarsal plate with continuous 6/0 or 7/0 absorbable suture. This covers the gold weight implant (Figure 7.6b).
- Close the skin with continuous 6/0 or 7/0 suture. Prescribe prophylactic systemic antibiotics for five days.

Complications – migration or extrusion may occur over several months. Resite the implant if necessary.

Direct brow lift (Figure 7.7)

The principle is to raise the brow by the excision of an ellipse of skin and frontalis

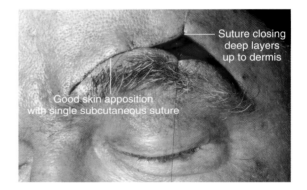

Figure 7.7   Deep sutures inserted in direct brow lift.

muscle, fixing it to the periosium of the forehead.

The *technique* is as follows:

- Mark the ellipse of tissue to be excised: mark first the superior border of the brow across its full width. Now manually lift the brow to the intended position, note the position, and allow the brow to fall again. Mark on the forehead skin the intended position of the superior border of the brow. Aim to over-correct slightly. Complete the marking of the ellipse with curved lines which join at the medial and lateral ends of the brow.
- Identify and mark the supraorbital notch through which the supraorbital nerve and vessels pass.

- Incise the ellipse of skin to the level of the frontalis muscle on the deep surface of the subcutaneous fat. Excise the ellipse of tissue. Special care is needed in the region of the supraorbital nerve and vessels.
- Close the deep layers with 4/0 nonabsorbable or long-acting absorbable sutures which include a deep bite through the periostium at the level of the superior wound edge. Omit the deep bite in the region of the supraorbital nerve and vessels. An extra row of more superficial subcutaneous sutures may be needed.
- Close the skin with a 4/0 monofilament subcuticular suture. Remove this at one week.

Complications – altered sensation in the forehead may occur due to damage to the supraorbital nerve. This may recover gradually over several months but it may be permanent. The position of the brow commonly droops again slightly in the weeks following surgery.

Corneal exposure

The risk factors for corneal exposure are well known: lid lag (inadequate eyelid closure), poor Bell's phenomenon, insensitive cornea and dry eye. Apart from release of a tight inferior rectus muscle to improve Bell's phenomenon and reduce upper lid retraction indirectly, the only surgical option in corneal exposure is to improve eyelid closure with or without overall reduction in the palpebral aperture. The latter may be achieved in either a vertical direction by lowering the upper lid and stabilising the lower lid or in a horizontal direction by approximating the lids at the inner or outer canthi.

Causes of inadequate eyelid closure

Select the surgical technique to improve corneal protection after analysing the causes of the inadequate eyelid closure. These can be conveniently classified as: orbicularis muscle functioning normally but normal lid closure prevented; orbicularis muscle not functioning normally; or eyelid defects.

Orbicularis muscle functioning normally

Tight skin, tight upper or lower lid retractors or tight conjunctiva prevent normal upper or lower lid movement and closure. Common causes are scarring and proptosis.

Tight skin – is due to scarring (or occasionally skin loss). Diffuse scarring is treated with a skin graft; linear scarring is treated with a z-plasty.

Tight upper or lower lid retractors – may be due to overcorrected ptosis or scarring. The retractors are recessed with either excision of Müller's muscle (simple recession is usually ineffective), or recession of the retractors themselves (levator aponeurosis or lower lid retractors). This is done through the anterior (skin) or the posterior (conjunctiva) approach. A spacer (e.g. sclera) is optional in the upper lid but is essential in the lower lid. Alternately, in the upper lid adjustable sutures may be used.

Tight conjunctiva – must be released and a graft of oral mucosa or hard palate inserted.

Proptosis – if severe (lid surgery alone is not effective) is treated with decompression of the medial wall and floor, and the lateral wall if necessary. A lateral tarsorrhaphy may be necessary in severe cases.

Orbicularis muscle not functioning normally

The commonest cause is facial palsy but patients who blink less than normal may have an added risk factor e.g. mental deficiency; comatose patients, especially those on ventilators; premature babies; etc.

Lid defects

For example, after tumour excision or trauma.

Surgical techniques in corneal protection

Skin grafting and z-plasty are described on p. 13, hard palate grafts on p. 30 and orbital decompression on p. 116. Surgical procedures in facial palsy are described above.

Upper lid retractor recession

The anterior approach is suitable for larger amounts of retraction; the posterior approach is better for smaller amounts. Since the posterior approach also results in a raised skin crease, it is preferable to restrict its use to bilateral cases.

The principle is that the levator aponeurosis and Müller's muscle are separated from the tarsal plate and recessed. Their position may be maintained with a spacer or with sutures, or left free.

The *technique* for the **anterior approach** is as follows (Figure 7.8a and b).

- Make an incision in the upper lid skin crease at the desired level. Deepen it through the orbicularis muscle to expose the full width of the tarsal plate.
- Dissect the skin and orbicularis muscle upwards for about 10–15mm to expose the anterior surface of the orbital septum. To confirm that it is the septum, press on the lower eyelid and look for the forward movement of the pre-aponeurotic fat pad behind it. Incise the septum horizontally to expose the pre-aponeurotic fat pad. Sweep the fat superiorly to expose the underlying levator aponeurosis and muscle.
- Dissect the levator aponeurosis and Müller's muscle from the superior border of the tarsal plate and continue the dissection between Müller's muscle and the conjunctiva as far as the superior conjunctival fornix. The upper lid retractors are now free of their inferior attachments and the tarsal plate can descend freely. If there is persistent retraction laterally, cut the lateral horn of the levator aponeurosis. If it still persists cut the lateral third of Whitnall's ligament and continue to free the tissues laterally until the retraction is overcome and there is a smooth curve to the lid. Decide whether a spacer is to be inserted to maintain the corrected lid position.
- *If a spacer is to be inserted* (Figure 7.8a), cut the spacer to the size required to allow adequate correction of the lid retraction. It is usually necessary to overcorrect the retraction by 2–3mm. Using 6/0 absorbable sutures, suture the edges of the spacer to the upper lid retractors (levator aponeurosis

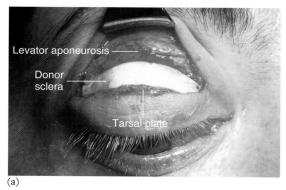
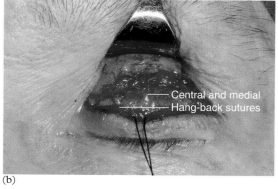

(a)   (b)

Figure 7.8   (a) Spacer of donor sclera placed between tarsal plate and levator aponeurosis, (b) upper lid retractors recessed and fixed with central and medical hang-back sutures.

and Müller's muscle) superiorly and to the superior tarsal plate border inferiorly.

- *If no spacer is to be used* (Figure 7.8b), estimate how much recession of the upper lid retractors is required and insert three 6/0 long-acting absorbable or nonabsorbable hang-back sutures. The lateral suture can be omitted if there was difficulty achieving satisfactory correction laterally.
- Close the lid with deep bites to create a skin crease. Insert a traction suture into the upper lid and tape it to the cheek until the first dressing.

The *technique* for the **posterior approach** is as follows (Figure 7.9a and b).

- Place a 4/0 stay suture into the centre of the tarsal plate close to the lid margin. Evert the lid over a Desmarres retractor. Make a short incision through the tarsal plate close to the superior border. An obvious surgical space – the post-aponeurotic space – is entered. Extend the incision medially and laterally, staying close to the superior border of the tarsal plate. The levator aponeurosis is the structure in the depths of the wound (see Figure 7.4).
- Pull down the lower wound edge which includes a strip of the superior tarsal plate and dissect between Müller's muscle

posteriorly and the levator aponeurosis anteriorly. Downward traction on Müller's muscle will expose a "white line" (Figure 7.9a) which is the edge of the levator aponeurosis folded on itself. Incise and turn down the levator aponeurosis for the full width of the tarsal incision to expose, but taking care not to damage the underlying orbicularis muscle (Figure 7.9b). Turn the lid back into its correct anatomical position and assess the correction of the retraction. An over-correction of 2–3mm is usually required. If it is inadequate, dissect superiorly between the levator aponeurosis and the orbicularis muscle for a few millimetres and reassess the lid position. Repeat this until adequate correction is achieved.

- Excise the narrow strip of superior tarsal plate – which is attached to the Müller's muscle. The retractors may be left free. Alternatively, suture them to the orbicularis muscle to fix their position.
- The conjunctiva does not need to be closed. Place a traction suture in the upper lid and tape it to the cheek until the first dressing.

Complications – the lid level, or the curve of the lid margin, may be incorrect. If there is no obvious cause, such as swelling, adjust the level early, within a week or so. If there

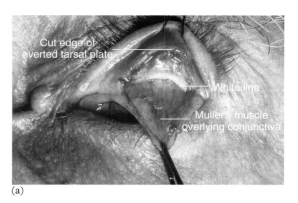

(a)

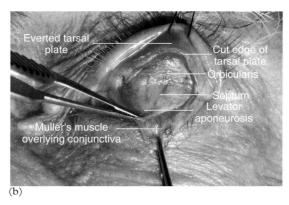

(b)

Figure 7.9   (a) Everted upper lid showing the 'white line' of the folded aponeurosis, (b) aponeurosis and septum exposed.

appears to be a probable cause, for example haematoma or swelling, and you think the lid may settle, wait then readjust the level, if necessary, at six months.

An inevitable side effect of an upper lid retractor recession by the posterior approach is that the skin crease is raised. Further surgery may be needed to restore symmetry of the upper lid skin creases and lid folds – either lowering the skin crease in the operated upper lid or raising the skin crease in the opposite upper lid.

Lower lid retractor recession (Figure 7.10)

The principle here is that the lower lid retractors are separated from the lower border of the tarsal plate and recessed. Their position is maintained with a spacer.

The *technique* is as follows:

- Place a stay suture through the lower tarsal plate close to the lid margin. Evert the lid over a Desmarres retractor.
- Make an incision through the conjunctiva close to the lower border of the tarsal plate. Carefully dissect the conjunctiva from the underlying, white, lower lid retractor layer, as far as the inferior fornix.
- Make an incision in the lower lid retractor layer to separate it from the lower border of the tarsal plate. Carefully dissect this layer from the underlying orbicularis muscle as far as the fornix, or until the retractors will recess inferiorly freely (Figure 7.10a). Cut an appropriate size of spacer to achieve slight overcorrection of the retraction – usually 2–3mm larger than the amount of retraction.

If hard palate is to be used as the spacer, rather than donor sclera, the conjunctiva and lower lid retractor layers can be dissected as one layer, and recessed together, because no conjunctival covering is needed. If sclera is to be used the layers must be dissected separately because a scleral spacer must be covered with conjunctiva.

- If donor sclera is to be used as the spacer suture the lower border of the sclera to the recessed lower lid retractor layer with 6/0 absorbable sutures (Figure 7.10b). Draw up the conjunctiva to cover the sclera and suture the superior border of the sclera, together with the edge of the conjunctiva,

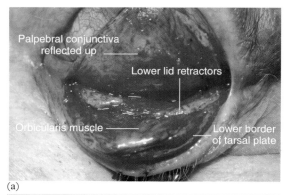

(a)

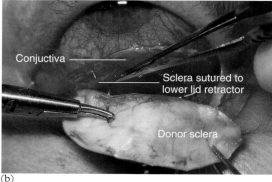

(b)

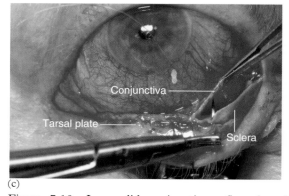

(c)

Figure 7.10 Lower lid conjunctiva reflected and lower lid retractors detached from tarsal plate, (b) spacer of donor sclera sutured to the lower lid retractors, (c) spacer covered with conjunctiva. All layers sutured to the lower border of the tarsal plate.

to the inferior border of the tarsal plate with a continuous 6/0 absorbable suture (Figure 7.10c).

- If a hard palate graft is to be used as the spacer recess the lower lid retractors and the conjunctiva together as one layer. Suture the lower edge of the graft to the recessed tissues and the superior edge to the inferior border of the tarsal plate using 6/0 absorbable sutures.

- Place three double-armed 4/0 sutures from the posterior aspect of the lid, through the graft to the skin and tie over small cotton wool bolsters. These sutures hold the layers together and are removed after a week. Place a traction suture in the lower lid and tape it to the forehead until the first dressing.

Complications – mild discomfort is common in the first few lays. The lid level will drop 1–2mm during the first few weeks.

Acknowledgement

Figures are modified from illustrations in Tyers AG, Collin JRO. *Colour Atlas of Ophthalmic Plastic Surgery, 2nd edn.* Oxford: Butterworth Heinemann, 2001.

Further reading

Adour KK, Diagnosis and management of facial palsy. *N Engl J Med* 1982; **307**:348–51.

Armstrong MWJ, Mountain RE, Murray JAM. Treatment of facial synkinesis and facial asymmetry with botulinum toxin type A following facial nerve palsy. *Clin Otolaryngol* 1996; **21**:15–20.

Cataland PJ, Bergstein MJ, Biller HF. Comprehensive management of the eye in facial paralysis. *Arch Otolaryngol – Head Neck Surg* 1995;**121**:81–6.

Crawford GJ, Collin, JRO, Moriarty PAJ. The correction of paralytic medial ectropion. *Br J Ophthalmol* 1984 **68**:639.

Kartush JM *et al.*, Early gold weight implantation for facial paralysis *Otolaryngol Head Neck Surg* 1990; **103**:1016–23.

Kirkness CM, Adams GG, Dilly PN, Lee JP. Botulinum toxin A-induced protective ptosis in corneal disease *Ophthalmology* 1988; **95**:473–80.

Lee OS. Operalion for correction of everted lacrimal puncta. *Am J Ophthalmol* 1951; **34**:575.

May M. Facial paralysis: differential diagnosis and indications for surgical therapy. *Clin Plast Surg* 1979; **6**:275–92.

May M. Croxson GR, Klein SR. Bell's palsy: management of sequelae using EMG, rehabilitation, botulinum toxin and surgery. *Am J Otol* 1989; **10**:220–9.

McCoy FJ, Goodman RC. The Crocodile Tear Syndrome. *Plast Reconstr Surg* 1979; **63**:58–62.

Olver JM, Fells P. Henderson's relief of eyelid retraction. *Eye* 1995; **9**:467–71.

Seiff SR, Chang J. The staged management of ophthalmic complications of facial nerve palsy. *Ophthal Plast Reconstr Surg* 1990; **9**:241–9.

Small RG. Surgery for upper eyelid retraction, three techniques. *Trans Am Ophthalmol Soc* 1995; **93**:353–69.

Tucker SM, Collin JRO. Repair of upper eyelid retraction: a comparison between adjustable and non-adjustable sutures. *Br J Ophthalmol* 1995; **79**:658–60.

Tyers AG, Collin JRO. *Colour Atlas of Ophthalmic Plastic Surgery, 2nd edn.* Oxford: Butterworth Heinemann, 2001.

8 Cosmetic surgery

Richard N Downes

Cosmetic surgery occupies an important part of the oculoplastic surgeon's workload. Increasingly patients request elective surgery to alter or improve their appearance. Patient selection, assessment, and surgical techniques differ in certain ways from non-aesthetic practice and appreciation of these differences is central to surgical success. Cosmetic surgery is both challenging and rewarding. The challenge posed is to effect the realistic expectations of the patient; it is with this goal in mind that the chapter has been written.

Patient evaluation

Patient selection and evaluation is of paramount importance in all branches of surgery; cosmetic surgery is no exception. A detailed history is essential. The patients' concerns and their expectations of surgery need to be established at the outset. Relevant past ophthalmic history should be taken including previous surgery, dry eyes or contact lens intolerance and general health problems, such as bleeding disorders, hypertension or diabetes. Similarly a past history of psychiatric or psychological disorders may prove important. Drug history is important with particular reference to anti-coagulants and aspirin, in addition to topical medication, and social and family history. Relevant factors such as outstanding or past litigation should also be noted.

Examination

Ask the patient to demonstrate what he/she is unhappy with and/or would like changed either in a mirror or with photographs. It is essential to note whether these concerns are appropriate and more importantly whether the expectations with regard to surgery realistic.

Examine the whole face for asymmetry, scarring etc. before examining specific areas of the face. It is important to remember that there are certain differences in facial structure between the female and male, such as brow and upper eyelid configuration, as well as racial variations. Surgery must always be planned with these variations in mind.

Examine the eyebrow configuration, position and symmetry. The male brow has a "T" shape configuration whilst that in the female is "Y" shaped. Assess the eyebrows for ptosis and symmetry, remembering that a patient may initially complain of eyelid ptosis when in fact the underlying problem is one of brow ptosis. The correct operation in this situation is a brow lift rather than blepharoplasty since the latter will if anything further accentuate the patient's problem. Brow ptosis and excess upper eyelid skin often co-exist; surgery should correct each of these components (Figures 8.1 and 8.2).

Examine the eyelids paying particular attention to the upper lid skin crease, lid contour and position, levator function, presence or absence of lagophthalmos and Bell's phenomenon. Assess the eyelids for

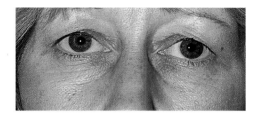

Figure 8.1 A patient with brow ptosis, excess upper eyelid skin and mid-face ptosis – pre-operatively.

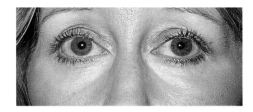

Figure 8.2 Post operative appearance of the same patient after face and brow lift, blepharoplasty and periocular laser resurfacing.

symmetry, excess lid tissue, i.e. is the problem one of dermatochalasis or blepharochalasis, and fat prolapse. Specifically examine for lower lid eyelid laxity. If this is present to any significant degree and lower lid blepharoplasty is contemplated then a lower lid tightening procedure may well be necessary. The lower lid skin is assessed for excess tissue, skin wrinkles and altered skin texture. If the latter is the case then periocular laser resurfacing may provide a better result with less risk of complications than skin excision. Is the patient suffering from festoons of excess lower lid skin? If so a variation in the surgical approach from conventional blepharoplasty may be needed.

Examine the rest of the face with particular attention to any scars, wrinkles and skin folds and generalised skin texture changes. It is important to document the patient's skin colouring and type which is best assessed using Fitzpatrick's classification. (Fitzpatrick described six skin types with types 1 and 2 representing a fair skin complexion, susceptible to sunburn, types 3 and 4 dark Mediterranean/Asian type of complexion, whilst 5 and 6 are deeply pigmented Afro-Caribbean skin types.)

Detailed ophthalmic examination must be undertaken. General ophthalmic examination should include best corrected visual acuity, assessment of ocular motility and slit lamp examination, the latter paying particular attention to the cornea and any evidence of dry eye syndrome, such as punctate corneal staining, a reduced tear film or break up time or an abnormal Schirmer's tear test.

Visual fields and any further specific tests are undertaken as necessary. Pre- and post operative photography is essential.

Patient discussion

The clinical findings and treatment options are explained in detail with the patient. Remember to be honest and realistic with regard to surgical outcomes as well as treatment limitations and complications. Ensure as much as you are able that the patient fully understands what treatment entails, that his/her expectations are realistic and that he/she is "psychologically fit" for any procedure. Always document what has been discussed.

Anaesthetic considerations

The anaesthetic options available for cosmetic surgery are local anaesthesia with or without sedation or general anaesthesia. Remember that surgery is elective and has been requested by the patient; it is incumbent upon the surgeon to ensure that any surgical treatment is as comfortable as possible.

Most procedures can be undertaken with local anaesthesia but supplementary intravenous anaesthesia provided by a trained anaesthetist should be considered in all cases, especially if the procedure is likely to be prolonged or the patient is apprehensive or nervous. Allow adequate time for the anaesthetic to take effect and ensure skin marking is undertaken before local infiltration. General anaesthesia should be considered if a number of areas of the face are operated on at the same time, the surgery is likely to be prolonged or at the patient's specific request. Supplementary local infiltrative anaesthesia is useful for haemostatic purposes as well as post operative analgesia even when general anaesthesia is the anaesthesia of choice.

Brow surgery

Brow ptosis generally results from ageing changes of the skin and soft tissues but may be secondary to other causes such as trauma or seventh nerve palsy. It is essential to examine for these and treat, as appropriate. Eyebrow ptosis which is characterised by inferior displacement of the brow, often below the orbital rim, is usually greatest laterally. If unilateral, the position is measured in relation to the opposite brow. If bilateral then the extent of ptosis is measured by comparing the difference in positions of marked fixed points on the brow medially, centrally and laterally when the brow is manually elevated to the desired position.

There are a number of approaches to surgical correction of brow ptosis.

Internal brow fixation (browpexy)

This is useful for the treatment of mild unilateral or bilateral, predominantly lateral, brow ptosis. It is often undertaken in conjunction with blepharoplasty.

The amount of brow lift is determined as outlined above. After a standard blepharoplasty upper lid skin crease incision, dissection is continued superiorly and laterally in the submuscular fascia plane over the orbital rim. Deep to the plane of dissection the brow fat pad is identified overlying the lateral orbital rim. This is excised on to periosteum. Between one and three 4/0 Prolene sutures are then used to fixate or plicate the brow to the periosteum in the desired position. The number of sutures used depends upon the

amount and extent of the brow lift required. The sutures are positioned 1cm apart and passed transcutaneously through the lower brow on to periosteum and horizontally through periosteum 1–1·5cm above the orbital rim. The suture is then passed back, again horizontally, through the brow muscle at the level of the transcutaneous suture avoiding superficial placement; the transcutaneous end of the suture is pulled through the brow tissue (but not the periosteum) and tied (Figure 8.3). This manoeuvre is a straightforward way of accurately positioning the suture with regard to both the periosteal and brow tissues. Additional sutures are used as required; if more than one suture is necessary then tying of the suture is best delayed until all sutures have been positioned. The height and curvature of the brow are assessed and adjusted as necessary. The skin incision is closed in the conventional way as for upper lid blepharoplasty.

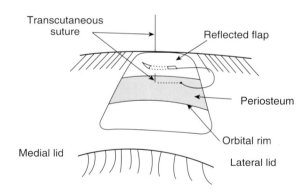

Figure 8.3 This demonstrates the horizontal periosteal suture, and return suture pass, before the transcutaneous suture is drawn through flap tissues only and tied.

Complications including skin dimpling, skin erosion and cheese-wiring of the sutures can occur with superficial placement. Contour and brow height abnormalities are seen with inappropriate suture placement. Recurrent brow ptosis may occur particularly if absorbable sutures have been used. Reduced eyelid elevation on upgaze is described which is an unavoidable limitation of the technique.

Direct brow lift (browplasty)

This procedure is particularly suitable for male patients with thick bushy eyebrows and receding hairlines (thereby masking brow scarring and avoiding coronal scarring), patients requiring a less extensive procedure and those with unilateral brow ptosis secondary to facial nerve palsy.

The extent of tissue excision is marked with the patient sitting upright aiming to position the scar within the upper row of brow hairs. The lower skin incision is made with the scalpel blade bevelled such that the incision is parallel to the hair shafts. This obviates transverse sectioning of the hair follicles thus minimising brow hair loss. Skin and subcutaneous tissue, with underlying orbicularis muscle as necessary, are excised taking care to identify and therefore avoid damage to the supraorbital neurovascular bundle. If surgery is undertaken for seventh nerve palsy then tissue excision down to the periosteum with deep fixation of brow tissue to periosteum using interrupted 4/0 Prolene sutures is necessary. The deeper tissues are closed with 4/0 or 5/0 Vicryl taking care to evert the skin edges prior to skin closure using a subcuticular 5/0 Prolene suture which is removed after five to seven days. This layered skin closure approach facilitates a thin flat scar.

Complications including loss of brow hair and/or an unsightly scar may result from poor surgical technique. An unacceptable brow position or contour is usually due to inappropriate marking. Permanent forehead parasthesia may occur with supraorbital nerve damage.

Mid forehead brow lift

This procedure is suitable for males with deep forehead furrows and excess forehead skin.

The forehead creases lying above the lateral brow are chosen as incision sites. Ideally the creases are at different levels over either brow. Following skin marking, skin, subcutaneous tissues and hypertrophic muscle are all excised as appropriate with layered wound closure as described in a direct brow lift.

The complications mainly relate to scarring and are minimised by careful surgical technique.

Temporal brow lift

This procedure is useful in patients with predominantly lateral brow ptosis. The incision site needs to be within the hairline and is therefore more appropriate for the female patient.

A 10–12cm vertical incision above the ear is made in the hair bearing scalp down to temporalis fascia. Blunt dissection towards the eyebrow initially at the plane of temporalis fascia then becoming more superficial over the scalp hairline (to minimise damage to superficial seventh branches) is undertaken. The flap is undermined onto the brow with excision of redundant scalp tissue followed by layered skin closure.

Complications include unacceptable elevation of the temporal hairline and local seventh nerve weakness if the facial nerve branches are damaged.

Coronal brow lift

This procedure is ideally suited to patients with a combination of brow ptosis, excessive forehead skin and soft tissue and a low non-receding hairline.

A bevelled high coronal incision is made within the hairline following the shape of the latter far enough posterior to position the subsequent scar 3–4cm posterior to the anterior hairline. The incision is angled to run parallel with the axis of the hair follicles down to periosteum. A forehead scalp flap is elevated using predominantly blunt dissection in the loose sub-galeal plane above the periosteum to within 2cm of the supraorbital rim centrally. Careful lateral dissection is undertaken avoiding seventh nerve branch damage. This is continued along the supraorbital rim with selective weakening surgery to the corrugator procerus and frontalis muscles avoiding damage to the supraorbital neurovascular bundles. A supraorbital periosteal incision may further enhance the procedure. Meticulous haemostasis throughout is essential before excision of excess flap tissue within the hairline. The wound is carefully closed in layers using deep 3/0 Vicryl and surgical staples or 4/0 Prolene, after placement of a supraorbital drain. The staples or sutures are removed seven to ten days post operatively.

Post operative haematoma leading to flap necrosis, localised sensory and motor nerve damage, hair loss and unacceptable scarring are all recognised complications, the majority of which can be avoided with careful surgical technique.

Endoscopic forehead and brow lift

This small incision technique is an alternative to the more extensive coronal brow lift. It facilitates brow elevation with coincident reduction of forehead creases whilst minimising scarring.

Two small vertical frontal incisions are made within the hairline on each side of the head down to bone followed by localised subperiosteal dissection, without endoscopic visualisation, backwards over the occiput, laterally over the parietal bone and towards the brow. Transverse temporal incisions, one on each side within the hairline, are then made on to deep temporalis fascia. These incisions are connected to the previously created subperiosteal dissection pockets, using blunt scissors, dissecting from the temporal incision centrally. The frontal and temporal spaces are joined to create an "optical cavity" thus facilitating further dissection using endoscopic control. This proceeds inferolaterally along the temporal line with subsequent fascial incision, facilitating adequate release of the lateral brow. Dissection with release of the periosteum, galea and depressor muscles is then undertaken.

The brows are now free for fixation which may be effected in a number of ways. The most common method is screw fixation whereby a screw is placed in each lateral frontal incision site at a predetermined distance from the anterior margin of the incision. A skin hook then pulls the periosteum margin posteriorly; the incision site is closed with staples or suture so that the screw is now at the anterior part of the wound and the forehead lifted and fixated by the predetermined amount. Additional fascial fixation may then be undertaken prior to skin closure using 4/0 Prolene or staples.

Complications are as for those described with bi-coronal brow lift technique, although with the exception of nerve damage, they occur less commonly.

Eyelid surgery

Upper eyelid blepharoplasty

Excess upper eyelid tissue and/or herniated orbital fat can be excised for functional or aesthetic reasons. In the former the excess tissues abut or overhang the lash margin, thus interfering with visual function. Significant coincidental brow ptosis must be repaired or it will be worsened by blepharoplasty.

The incision is marked with the patient sitting up. A line is drawn along the skin crease starting above the superior punctum extending to the lateral canthus and then sloping upwards 1–1·5cm from the lateral canthus in a natural skin crease (Figure 8.4). The skin above this area is pinched vertically using fine tooth forceps, the lower jaw of which is positioned on the marked line such that excess skin is eliminated and the lids

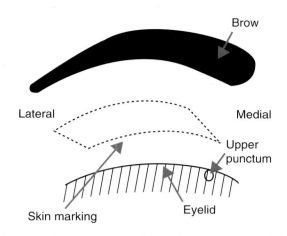

Figure 8.4 Skin marking for upper eyelid blepharoplasty.

just touch with passive lid closure. The position of the superior jaw of the forceps is marked. This method of marking is repeated nasally and temporally and the marks joined with similar preparation of the other eyelid remembering to aim for a symmetric post operative appearance. If local infiltrative anaesthesia is used it is injected at this stage.

The skin is incised with a scalpel along the marked line and excised from the underlying orbicularis. A strip of orbicularis may be removed if the muscle is felt to be bulky or significant skin excision has been undertaken. Orbital fat excision is undertaken if appropriate. Excess upper lid fat is usually confined to the central and medial areas of the eyelid. An apparent lateral protrusion is invariably a prolapsed lacrimal gland which should not be excised but rather repositioned using plicating sutures between the anterior gland capsule and supraorbital rim. Fat prolapse is facilitated by incision through the orbicularis and underlying fat capsule; gentle pressure on the globe via the lower lid enhances fat prolapse. It is essential that the fat is handled carefully and gently to avoid unnecessary traction on posterior orbital fat and associated blood vessels. The excess fat to be removed is clamped and excised with cautery to the excision stump. Meticulous care is necessary throughout with particular regard to haemostasis.

If excess medial canthal skin is present then this is excised by extension of the medial incision superiorly with excision of redundant overlying skin. It is not necessary to close either orbital septum or the deeper layers of the eyelid. The skin is sutured with an over and over 6/0 Prolene centrally reinforced with individual sutures at the medial and lateral angulation, which are removed four to five days post operatively.

To minimise post operative bruising and facilitate healing, ice-packs are applied for 24 hours post operatively. The vision is checked hourly for the first four hours post operatively. The patient is advised to report sudden orbital pain or loss of vision immediately.

Lower eyelid blepharoplasty

Lower eyelid blepharoplasty is generally undertaken for cosmetic purposes. Three different approaches are described.

Anterior approach blepharoplasty

Anterior approach blepharoplasty is indicated in patients with excess lower eyelid skin and fat prolapse.

Technique – a subciliary incision is marked 1–2mm below the lash line starting inferior to the punctum, running across the lid to the lateral canthus and extending straight laterally for up to 1cm in the line of a natural skin crease (Figure 8.5). The skin is incised with a scalpel and deepened centrally on to the tarsus. A skin muscle flap is initially fashioned and elevated off the tarsus and septum, then extended laterally and medially using scissors. A 4/0 traction suture through the tarsus superior to the incision site allows controlled eyelid traction upwards which facilitates flap dissection. Dissection is continued inferiorly in the suborbicularis plane to the orbital rim, thereby exposing orbital septum throughout the lower eyelid. Orbital fat lies deep to the orbital septum and is prolapsed when the

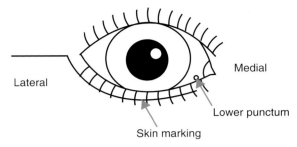

Figure 8.5 Skin marking for lower eyelid blepharoplasty.

septum is opened across the horizontal length of the eyelid. The fat is localised in three fat pads temporally, centrally and nasally and careful graded excision of the fat starting temporally and proceeding medially is undertaken with meticulous haemostasis, again avoiding unnecessary posterior traction. The skin muscle flap is swept superiorly on maximal stretch (with the patient looking up and the mouth open), excess flap tissue is marked and redundant skin and muscle then excised. The wound is closed with a single over and over 6/0 Prolene suture along the lid incision and interrupted 6/0 sutures laterally.

In cases with co-existent lid laxity a horizontal lid shortening procedure, in the form of either a lateral full thickness pentagon lid excision or lateral canthal sling, is undertaken before skin and muscle excision.

Similarly if co-existent mid-face ptosis is present then a mid-facelift may be necessary. Surgery to correct this should immediately precede any lid shortening procedure if this surgical combination is undertaken. The skin muscle flap is retracted downwards to expose the inferior orbital rim. Various techniques have been described to undermine and elevate the cheek, or mid-face, tissues. In the SOOF (suborbital orbicularis oculi fat) lift a cheek flap is raised at the periosteal level; alternatively a subperiosteal flap may be fashioned. With either approach, dissection is continued inferiorly to the level where the cheek bone ends and nasally towards the nasolabial fold, taking care to avoid infraorbital

nerve damage. With the subperiosteal approach the periosteum is incised 2–3mm below the orbital rim with inferior dissection and periosteal release such that the cheek flap is freely elevated. The latter is attached superiorly to the periosteum of the lateral orbital wall and orbital rim with interrupted 4/0 Prolene such that the ptotic cheek is lifted upwards and laterally. Excess skin and muscle are excised and the skin closed as for conventional blepharoplasty.

Ice packs are applied in the immediate post operative period with regular assessment of the vision as with upper lid blepharoplasty.

Transconjunctival blepharoplasty

Transconjunctival blepharoplasty is indicated in patients with fat prolapse but without excess skin.

The lower eyelid is infiltrated with local anaesthesia subcutaneously and trans-conjunctivally down to the orbital rim. A marginal traction suture is placed and the lid everted over a Desmarres retractor. The conjunctiva is incised 4mm below the inferior tarsal margin, extending the width of the eyelid, using scissors, cutting cautery or laser. The incision is carried through the deeper tissues until fat is exposed. The incision is held open with outward and downward traction which facilitates fat exposure. The fat capsule is incised with judicious fat excision from the three fat pads as appropriate and meticulous haemostasis, again avoiding unnecessary posterior fat traction. The conjunctival incision can either be left unsutured or closed with interrupted 6/0 absorbable sutures.

Post operatively ice packs are applied with regular visual assessment as for conventional blepharoplasty.

External direct lower eyelid blepharoplasty

This procedure is reserved for excision of significant lower eyelid tissue in the form of festoons.

The skin and excess underlying tissues to be excised are outlined taking care to position the excision symmetrically and, if possible, in a co-existent lid crease in the area overlying the inferior orbital rim. The skin and deeper tissues are incised followed by excision of all excess tissue using scissors. Haemostasis is secured. Layered closure with careful skin margin approximation using a 6/0 subcuticular Prolene suture is undertaken which is removed five to seven days post operatively.

Blepharoplasty complications

Blindness is described as occurring in between 1:10 000 and 1:40 000 cases. It only occurs when the orbital compartment is entered with fat excision and is thought to be related to traction on the posterior orbital vessels with subsequent orbital haemorrhage.

Diplopia is an uncommon complication of blepharoplasty usually related to damage to the inferior oblique muscle.

Ptosis may occur transiently or permanently. It is caused by either direct damage or significant stretching of the levator muscle.

Inadequate or excessive skin excision may result in a number of complications. If excess upper lid skin is excised lagophthalmos results which may or may not be a permanent feature. More marked excess upper lid skin excision may result in frank lid margin rotation and ectropion. Excess skin removal from the lower lid can result in rounding of the lateral canthal region with enhancement of scleral show and frank lid margin ectropion or lid retraction. Excess skin removal is the commonest significant complication following blepharoplasty. The abnormal lid position may respond to vigorous regular lid massage but often recourse to revisionary lid surgery is necessary. Inadequate skin removal requires further skin excision.

Fat excision may be inadequate or excessive. Significant excess fat excision will result in a hollowed out appearance particularly apparent in the lower lid. Surgery in the form of suborbicularis oculi fat transposition may be necessary to rectify this asymmetry. If fat excision has been limited then further fat removal may be necessary.

Lid asymmetry as a consequence of improperly positioned incisions is described. The most noticeable asymmetry relates to asymmetric skin crease positions which if unacceptable will require revisionary surgery.

Lasers in oculoplastic surgery

The use of lasers in oculoplastic surgery has become increasingly widespread of late. Two lasers are at present pre-eminent in the field; the carbon dioxide and more recently erbium YAG lasers. The basic principle for all these lasers is that of delivering high laser energy in short pulses or bursts, thus maximising tissue ablation whilst minimising adjacent thermal damage and hence scarring. The current lasers produce these short burst effects either by the provision of a super or ultra pulse pattern such as the Coherent CO_2 laser or Erbium YAG or a continuous wave laser which is interrupted by a rapidly moving mechanical system such as the Sharplan laser.

A number of carbon dioxide laser systems are currently available for oculoplastic surgery. Carbon dioxide lasers have both tissue ablative and haemostatic properties which make them ideally suited for both incisional and resurfacing surgery.

The Erbium YAG laser delivers increased tissue ablation with co-incidental reduction of adjacent thermal damage when compared to the carbon dioxide laser. This results in reduced tissue damage, erythema and post operative inflammation. The major disadvantages of the erbium YAG are lack of coagulation, so that it is not suitable for incisional surgery, and lack of contractile effect when used for resurfacing which may be important in the maintenance of medium to long term effects.

Skin resurfacing

Laser skin resurfacing is used to smooth facial skin and reduce wrinkles or rhytides. Dynamic rhytides resulting from underlying muscle activity, i.e. glabellar folds do not respond as well as static rhytides, i.e. periocular folds caused by ageing and ultraviolet exposure. The technique of laser skin resurfacing results in vaporisation of the epidermis and upper dermal layers with subsequent repair resulting in an improved cosmetic appearance. This relatively precise skin ablation with reduced thermal damage results in a more reproducible and superior result than alternative techniques such as dermabrasion or chemical peels.

Patients for laser resurfacing should be carefully selected and understand the aims and limitations of laser treatment. A thorough history with particular emphasis upon the use of topical skin preparations, allergies and sensitivities and previous herpetic infections is taken. Fair skinned patients (Fitzpatrick grades 1 and 2) are ideal for resurfacing whereas darker skinned individuals (Fitzpatrick grades 3 and 4) run a risk of post laser hyperpigmentation and should be approached cautiously. Laser resurfacing is contra-indicated in patients with deeply pigmented skin (Fitzpatrick grades 5 and 6). Pre-operative photographs with detailed diagrams and sketches are mandatory.

Technique of carbon dioxide laser resurfacing

Pre-operative skin preparation may be necessary in certain patients. Prophylactic anti-virals, i.e. Zovirax and oral antibiotics are frequently used and started 24 hours pre-operatively. If limited areas are being resurfaced, i.e. periocular or perioral regions only, then local anaesthesia, either infiltrative or regional nerve blocks, with or without intravenous sedation is used. Full face resurfacing is best undertaken using local anaesthesia and sedation or general anaesthesia.

Laser safety precautions must always be observed which include protection of areas not being treated with wet swabs and/or protective eye shields. Anaesthetic equipment if used, must be protected using silver foil around the exposed endotracheal tube and connection and all theatre staff, including the surgeon, must wear protective goggles.

Techniques for resurfacing vary greatly from one surgeon to the next but all adhere to certain basic tenets. The skin thickness varies considerably over different parts of the face with the periocular skin being the thinnest and skin over the cheek and chin the thickest. In order to achieve a similar improvement in each area more laser treatment or resculpting is necessary with the thickest tissues.

The skin is thoroughly cleansed with saline and dried. The area of treatment is outlined and any deep wrinkles individually marked. The laser pattern and power are set, the laser tested and treatment commenced. The initial treatment centres on the individual wrinkles or scars outlined, with treatment to the shoulders or elevated areas adjacent to the deeper wrinkle or scar. The ablated debris is removed with saline soaked gauze swabs. Confluent laser passes are then made over the entire region or regions to be treated, taking care to avoid significant overlap of the laser pattern. The number of passes with the laser is dependent on the region of skin treated and the laser characteristics. Usually 1–2 passes are all that is required when treating periocular skin whilst 2–4 passes may be necessary in areas of thicker skin such as the forehead, cheeks or chin. All desiccated tissue must be carefully wiped away with saline swabs after each pass (Figure 8.6). Assessment of the depth of treatment is facilitated by recognised colour changes occurring in the tissues.

Complete epithelial removal results in a pinkish appearance; treatment to the papillary dermal layer correlates with a yellow/orange coloration whilst deeper reticular dermal ablation is characterised by a chamois leather or white appearance. Treatment should stop at this latter stage as deeper laser treatment may well lead to hypertrophic scarring.

It is important to avoid a frank demarcation line between areas of treated and untreated facial skin. This is facilitated by feathering or blending of the adjacent areas whereby laser treatment using reduced power and wider spacing is undertaken.

Post operatively it is essential to keep the treated area moist or covered at all times until re-epithelialisation has occurred which is usually complete within five to seven days. Many techniques have been described ranging from regular applications of aqueous cream and cleansing through to custom designed dressings.

After re-epithelialisation it is again important to keep the treated area moist. Most patients elect to use a combined moisturising concealer preparation until the erythematous phase of the treatment (lasting anything up to three months from the time of laser treatment) has settled. It is essential that the patient treats the newly resurfaced skin very carefully, rather like a baby's skin. Direct sunlight must be avoided and a sunblock preparation always used when outdoors, ideally long term.

Most post operative problems, assuming that laser treatment has been appropriately undertaken, result from poor skin care. Redness or erythema is to be expected and may take up to three months or more to settle. Hyper- or rarely hypo-pigmentation can occasionally occur. The former can be managed with topical skin bleaching agents or steroid preparations but there is relatively little that can be offered for hypo-pigmentation.

Incisional surgery

The carbon dioxide laser can be used for tissue cutting as in blepharoplasty. The improved haemostasis allows for better visualisation during surgery, more rapid surgery and less post operative bruising and discomfort. Incisional laser surgery is particularly useful in transconjunctival blepharoplasties. Fat excision can be more carefully controlled with regard to both the amount of tissue excised and haemostasis at excision, without requirement for clamping of the fat to be excised. The possibility of undue posterior traction on the fat is therefore virtually abolished; the latter may well prove to be an important advantage of laser over conventional techniques. When transconjunctival blepharoplasty is combined with periocular resurfacing, very acceptable results can be achieved in patients with general wrinkling and skin laxity, and associated fat prolapse, without the complications normally associated with conventional subciliary blepharoplasty and skin excision.

Erbium YAG laser

The principles of resurfacing with the erbium YAG laser are broadly similar to those outlined using the carbon dioxide laser. The skin change colours characteristic of carbon dioxide laser resurfacing, are not seen with the erbium YAG. Break through punctate bleeding occurs as a consequence of lack of coagulation which,

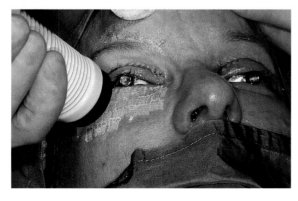

Figure 8.6   Periocular laser resurfacing with CO_2 laser.

although useful in assessing the depth of treatment, is a limiting factor when undertaking deeper resurfacing. The recovery, in particular the duration of post operative erythema, with erbium YAG resurfacing is significantly reduced compared to the carbon dioxide laser and this appears to be its major advantage.

At the present time the carbon dioxide and erbium YAG lasers should be considered as complementary. As such the oculoplastic surgeon should be familiar with and have access to both systems.

Further reading

Alster TS, Apfelberg DB. *Cosmetic Laser Surgery* (1st ed.) New York: Wiley-Liss Inc, 1996.

Collin JRO. *A Manual of Systematic Eyelid Surgery* (2nd ed.) Oxford: Butterworth-Heinemann, 1989.

De Mere M, Wood T, Austin W. Eye Complications with Blepharoplasty or Other Eyelid Surgery. A National Survey. *Plast Reconstr Surg* 1974; **53**:634–7.

McCord Jr CD, Tanenbaum M, Nunery WR. *Oculoplastic Surgery* (3rd ed.) New York: Raven Press, 1995.

Putterman AM. *Cosmetic Oculoplastic Surgery* (3rd ed.) Philadelphia: WB Saunders Company, 1999.

9 Socket surgery

Carole A Jones

The absence or loss of an eye is of enormous psychological significance to any patient. Socket surgery is directed at enabling the patient to wear a comfortable cosmetic ocular prosthesis which is stable and free from discharge. Removal of the eye and or orbital tissues may be necessary as a result of trauma, infection, tumour, the consequence of a painful eye or to remove a cosmetically unattractive globe. Depending upon the nature of the pathology the globe should be removed by evisceration, enucleation or exenteration.

Evisceration

The procedure involves the removal of ocular contents, retaining the scleral coat (Figure 9.1). There is no involvement of the meninges or optic nerves so little risk of backward spread of infection. The operation is less traumatic than enucleation and normally results in minimal bleeding; this may be of particular significance in the presence of orbital inflammation. The ocular remnant is fully mobile and there is less late orbital fat atrophy.

A contra-indication to evisceration is the theoretical risk of subsequent sympathetic uveitis although if uveal tissue is carefully removed the incidence of this condition appears extremely low. This surgery should not be performed when there is a risk of local tumour recurrence or when an intraocular tumour cannot be excluded. Furthermore, histological assessment of the specimens obtained at the time of evisceration are difficult to interpret.

Evisceration can be performed with or without keratectomy. The ocular contents are evacuated with an evisceration spoon introduced into the supra-choroidal space. Haemostasis is achieved by packing, and all remnants of uveal tissue should be carefully removed. The scleral cavity can be swabbed with dressed orange sticks moistened with absolute alcohol.

In the presence of suppuration the scleral envelope may be packed open and allowed to heal by secondary intention. In primary closure, if keratectomy has been performed, two triangles of sclera are excised at 9 and 3 o'clock allowing secure closure over an implant. The evisceration is completed by a three layered closure, sclera, Tenon's capsule and finally conjunctiva, using 5/0 Vicryl (Figure 9.1).

Enucleation

This procedure (Figure 9.2) involves the removal of the entire globe by severing the attachments of the extra-ocular muscles and optic nerves. This is the technique of choice in the presence of an intra-ocular tumour as histological specimens are easily obtained. There is no associated risk of sympathetic ophthalmitis. The surgery requires care to

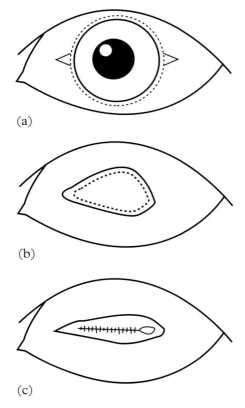

(a)

(b)

(c)

Figure 9.1 Evisceration. (a) 360° peritomy, anterior chamber opened, cornea removed, two triangles of sclera excised at 3 and 9 o'clock; (b) evisceration spoon used to remove contents of globe, scleral shell cleaned; (c) scleral shell closed with 5/0 Vicryl.

prevent socket contracture or late post operative fat atrophy.

A 360° peritomy is made in the conjunctiva and Tenon's capsule is carefully separated from the globe. The four rectus muscles are identified and tagged with double ended 5/0 Vicryl sutures. The two oblique muscles are cut or the inferior oblique may be tagged and sutured to the inferior border of the lateral rectus, 10mm posterior to its free edge. The optic nerve is sectioned with scissors or a snare. The globe is removed and the socket packed, using gauze soaked in iced saline to achieve haemostasis.

An ocular implant is generally inserted, either within Tenon's capsule or posterior to the posterior part of Tenon's capsule. Deep

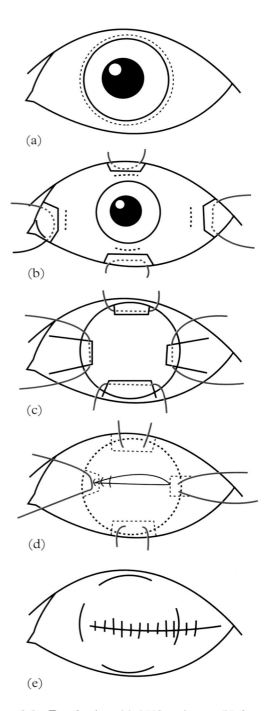

(a)

(b)

(c)

(d)

(e)

Figure 9.2 Enucleation. (a) 360° peritomy; (b) four rectus muscles disinserted, oblique muscles cut, optic nerve divided, globe removed; (c) wrapped spherical orbital implant inserted, rectus muscles saturated to implant; (d) tenons capsule closed, muscle sutures brought out through conjunctiva; (e) conjunctiva closed.

placement of the orbital implant in this site posterior to Tenon's capsule allows a larger volume to be implanted and reduces the incidence of implant migration or extrusion. The orbital implant may be of inert material, for example silicone ball or one that allows fibrovascular ingrowth, for example Medpor and Hydroxyapatite. Implants are wrapped in a synthetic mesh or donor sclera. The four rectus muscles are attached to the implant. The superior rectus should not be placed too anteriorly to minimise the incidence of upper lid retraction or ptosis. When using Hydoxyapatite, holes should be made in the wrap to allow the attachment of the extra ocular muscles and to facilitate fibro-vascular ingrowth. Muscle sutures are then placed through the conjunctival fornices to improve prosthesis mobility. Tenon's capsule and conjunctiva are closed carefully in two layers. A conformer, with a large central drainage hole should be inserted post operatively and left in place until a prosthesis is fitted at approximately six weeks.

Enucleation is not appropriate in the presence of endophthalmitis nor where a malignant tumour may have spread to extra-ocular structures. In this case an exenteration should be performed. An orbital implant is normally inserted at the time of primary enucleation but may be avoided in the presence of intraocular malignancy or in a very inflamed orbit where the incidence of post operative extrusion is high.

Exenteration

This involves the total excision of the orbital contents, with or without the removal of the eyelids. Indications for this surgery are advanced malignancy, either of the eyelid, the globe or surrounding adnexal structures. The extent of the procedure depends upon the size and extent of the tumour. If the tumour of the globe does not involve the eyelid skin the lids may be retained but they must be sacrificed in the presence of an extensive skin tumour.

An elliptical incision is made through the skin and deep tissues to the bone of the orbital rim. The periosteum is separated from the bony orbit; the trochlea, medial and lateral canthal tendons are detached. The apical structures, including the optic nerve, are cut and the orbital contents are removed within the periosteum. The orbit may be allowed to heal by granulation or a split skin graft used to line the bony cavity.

If the eyelid skin is to be preserved the periorbital skin is undermined, the lid margins are sacrificed and the resultant skin edges sutured together. The dead space behind the skin is gradually obliterated as the skin adheres to the bony orbit. Any attempt to replace the volume within the orbit using a thick skin flap or temporalis muscle may make the detection of local recurrences more difficult.

Orbital implants

When the globe is removed its volume cannot be replaced solely with an ocular prosthesis. By replacing orbital volume in the form of a orbital implant a light artificial eye can be fitted.

Box 9.1 Calculation of implant volume

Globe volume	= 8ml
Implant volume	= globe volume – prosthesis volume
	= 8ml – 2ml
Ideal implant volume	= 6ml

Many shapes have been suggested but a sphere is routinely used as it has the maximum volume for a given surface area. An 18mm sphere has a volume of 3ml and when wrapped this increases to 4ml. Studies have shown that patients may require larger volume. More recently a conoid shape with a flat front surface has been suggested.

In 1885 Mules first suggested the insertion of a glass ball into the scleral cup. Subsequently inert materials such as silicone and methyl methacrylate have been developed. More recently, a natural component of coral reefs known as porous hydroxyapatite has proved to be an ideal implant material. This allows fibro-vascular ingrowth, the implant becoming fully integrated rather than forming a sequestrated foreign body, as was the case with inert ball implants. Synthetic and cheaper forms of hydroxyapatite and other integrateable materials such as Medpor (porous polyethylene) are also now available.

Orbital implants are generally wrapped to allow ease of placement and to allow attachment of the extra-ocular muscles. Inert implants are best inserted posterior to Tenon's capsule whilst hydroxyapatite should be inserted within Tenon's capsule.

The aim of orbital implantation is to increase orbital volume and promote prosthesis mobility. It is essential that the orbital implant is stable and does not extrude. Until recently attempts to improve mobility in the form of partially exposed peg-type

---

Box 9.2 Classification of materials used in orbital implants

Orbital implant materials:
- Synthetic – silicone, Medpor
- Naturally occurring – Hydroxyapatite
- Autogenous – dermofat graft

Wrapping materials:
- Synthetic – Gortex, Vicryl mesh
- Homologous – fascia lata, dura, sclera
- Autogenous – temporalis fascia, fascia lata

---

implants have led to a high extrusion rate. Hydroxyapatite, as it becomes fully integrated with fibro-vascular ingrowth, allows direct coupling of the orbital implant and prosthesis. Following implantation and integration of the Hydroxyapatite a drill hole is placed, into which a peg can be inserted. This can be made to fit a depression in the artificial eye which can further improve prosthesis mobility although it is not always necessary.

Complications of orbital implants

Extrusion of implant

- Early (in the first six weeks)
  - Inadequate suturing of Tenon's capsule and conjunctiva
  - Infection
  - Too large an orbital implant
- Late
  - Chronic infection
  - Pressure necrosis
  - Poorly fitted prosthesis
  - Inappropriate orbital implant.

Early extrusion may be controlled with resuturing of Tenon's capsule and conjunctiva. Chronic extrusion requires patching the extruded area with sclera or fascia lata. In the presence of infection removal of the orbital implant may be necessary.

Migration of the implant

Here the implant migrates outside the muscle cone leading to decentration of the artificial eye. This requires removal and secondary implantation.

Dermis fat grafts

In certain circumstances, such as following implant extrusion, it may be inappropriate to reinsert a foreign body into the orbit. A useful autogenous graft to replace orbital volume, and if necessary to increase socket lining, is de-epithelialised dermofat. Dermofat grafts do not fare well in extensively traumatised sockets nor in severely contracted sockets with poor vascularity.

De-epithelialised dermofat is harvested from a donor site, generally the upper outer quadrant of the buttocks. Here, even in thin individuals, a moderate degree of fat exists and the donor site is easily hidden.

A horizontal ellipse is marked of appropriate size allowing a circle of 2·5cm diameter of dermis with attached fat of 3–4cm in depth to be harvested. The size of the graft should be tailored to the amount of orbital replacement required, allowing for an expected shrinkage of at least 25%. One per cent lignocaine with adrenaline is injected superficially into the dermis to allow a split skin graft to be taken. Once the epithelium has been removed in this way the ellipse of dermis, with attached fat to a depth up to twice the diameter of the dermis, is removed. 3·0 catgut is used to close the fat and 4·0 black silk or nylon to close the skin. A pressure dressing should be applied and the patient should be advised not to soak the wound in a bath until it is fully healed.

The socket is prepared as for the insertion of other orbital implants. All measures to encourage vascularity of the graft are taken. These include opening Tenon's capsule to encourage ingrowth of blood vessels, attachment of four rectus muscles to the graft and suturing the conjunctiva and Tenon's capsule to the surface of the graft. If muscles cannot be identified the subconjunctival fibrous tissue should be opened and sutured to the graft as this will contain the muscle insertions. Particular care should be paid to haemostasis and minimal handling of the graft to maximise graft survival.

Complications

Donor site

- Wound dehiscence – avoid physical activity and soaking of the skin edges. Sutures can be left in for up to 3 weeks and removed in stages.
- Wound infection – this is minimised by the routine use of post operative systemic antibiotics.

By harvesting dermofat from the upper outer buttocks post operative discomfort and unsightly scarring are minimised.

Socket

- Early
  - Graft failure, partial.
    Here, central necrosis and ulceration occurs as vascularisation of the centre of the graft is delayed. This area frequently heals with time or if necessary the central avascular ulcer can be excised and the edges sutured directly.
  - Graft failure, total.
    Here, shrinkage and pallor of the graft occurs within the first few weeks following the operation. If appropriate, repeated surgery may be necessary.
  - Infection – minimised by routine post operative systemic antibiotics.

- Late
  - Residual epithelium – if skin and conjunctiva co-exist this can be associated with a creamy discharge from the socket which may require removal of the residual skin epithelium.
  - Hair growth – hair may appear on the surface of the graft. This often disappears within a period of months, if not the hair can be removed by electrolysis.
  - Granuloma formation – post operative granulomas may need to be removed surgically.

The volume deficient socket (post-enucleation socket syndrome)

Main features

- Enophthalmus
- Ptosis
- Deep upper lid sulcus
- Lax lower lid.

With the loss of the globe and post operative fat atrophy enophthalmos of the prosthesis occurs. Attempts to improve this by fitting a larger artificial eye lead to lower lid laxity and downward displacement of the lower lid with the loss of the inferior fornix and associated deepening of the upper lid sulcus. The prosthesis no longer provides an adequate fulcrum for the levator muscle so ptosis results. In some cases retraction of the upper lid rather than ptosis is seen as a feature of a volume deficient socket. This is due to retraction of the levator complex with posterior rotation of the orbital contents. This further deepens the superior sulcus and there is associated forward redistribution of the orbital fat and upward displacement of the inferior rectus, all resulting in a backwards tilt of the prosthesis.

Management of post-enucleation socket syndrome

Each of the features of the post enucleation syndrome should be assessed:

- Enophthalmos – evident clinically but may be quantified using exophthalmometry measurements.
- Ptosis – assessment of the degree of ptosis and amount of levator function is necessary. The margin reflex distance and skin crease should be recorded. The tarsoconjunctival surface should also be examined.
- Deep upper lid sulcus – evident as hollowing above the upper lid.

- Lower lid laxity – the degree of lower lid laxity and the strength of the medial canthal tendon should be assessed. The inferior fornix depth should be reviewed as lid laxity may be associated with a shallow inferior fornix.

To correct the features of the volume deficient socket its components must be managed in an appropriate order. Volume replacement is the primary requirement followed by the surgical correction of the lax lower lid and shallowing of the inferior fornix. Finally, once all other features have been resolved, any residual ptosis can be addressed following the principles described in ptosis surgery elsewhere.

By supplementing orbital volume and correcting enophthalmos, a lighter well-positioned prosthesis will provide a better fulcrum for levator. The prosthesis becomes more stable and cosmetically acceptable.

- *Replacement of orbital volume with an orbital implant.* Where an inadequate orbital implant exists this should be replaced with a larger implant. The details of this procedure are covered in the section on enucleation (page 93). In the presence of a previously extruded orbital implant, autogenous material such as dermofat should be employed, as described earlier.
- *Replacement of orbital volume with sub-periosteal implant.* Using a subciliary blepharoplasty approach a skin and muscle flap is raised to expose the inferior orbital rim. The periosteum is incised and elevated to reveal the orbital floor. A flat topped, wedge shaped block of silicone or Medpor is inserted deep into the periosteum this acts to elevate the orbital contents, displacing them superiorly and anteriorly. The periosteum is closed with 4/0 Vicryl and the skin and muscle flap sutured using 6/0 black silk.
- *Horizontal lid laxity.* A full thickness lid resection or lateral tarsal strip should

be undertaken. These procedures are described in Chapter 3.

- *Lower lid fascial sling.* If the medial canthal tendon is lax, lateral canthal tightening will result in the lateral displacement of the inferior punctum. This can be avoided using a fascialata sling between the medial and lateral canthal tendons. Such a sling will support a heavy prosthesis if necessary. Fascia lata is harvested as for brow suspension. Stored fascia lata can be used as an alternative material.

  Three incisions are made in the lower lid. A vertical medial incision over the medial canthal tendon, a central subciliary incision and a lateral horizontal incision which overlies the lateral orbital rim and exposes the lateral canthal tendon. A 3mm wide strip of facia, cut parallel to the line of the collagen fibres, is used. It is looped over the medial canthal tendon and sutured to itself. Using a Wright's fascial needle, introduced from the central subciliary incision, the free end of fascia is drawn laterally deep to orbicularis and pulled out through the central lid incision.

  The fascia should pass deep into the orbicularis but superficial to the tarsal plate. The Wright's needle is reinserted from the lateral canthal incision and the fascia drawn further laterally.

  Finally the free lateral end of the fascia is passed through the upper limb of the lateral canthal tendon and sutured to the orbital periosteum. Alternatively burr holes can be made in the lateral wall and the fascia anchored in this way.

- *Shallowing of the inferior fornix.* This may occur if the fornix is not well maintained in the early post operative period or forward migration of the orbital implant occurs. Symblepharon may develop with abnormal adhesion between the bulbar and palpebral conjunctiva. A heavy prosthesis that rests on the lower lid, stretching it, may lead to further shallowing of the inferior fornix. It can be treated by

- *Removal of the cause.* For example, reposition intra-orbital implant.

- *Reconstitution of the inferior fornix.* Commonly some element of cicatrisation occurs but if the conjunctiva is adequate the inferior fornix can be reformed using fornix deepening sutures attached to the orbital rim. If cicatrisation exists the conjunctiva of the inferior fornix is opened and dissection continued down to the orbital rim. Any scar tissue should be excised. A buccal mucous membrane graft is inserted deep within the inferior fornix and sutured to the conjunctival edges. A silicone rod or gutter is held in the inferior fornix and 4/0 nylon sutures attached to the gutter are passed through the inferior periosteum to emerge through the skin well below the lid margin. These sutures are tied on the skin surface over bolsters. The sutures are left in place for three weeks. Fornix deepening can be coupled with lid shortening procedures.

- *Ptosis.* Once adequate volume replacement has been achieved a better fitting artificial eye re-establishes the normal fulcrum for levator complex and ptosis improves. Any residual ptosis may be due to damage of the levator complex at the time of injury or surgery and correction is dependent upon the degree of levator function. With a good levator function a levator resection should be performed, if the levator function is poor a brow suspension procedure is a more appropriate operation. It is preferable to avoid any operation which will interfere with the tarso-conjunctiva of the upper lid such as Fasanella Servat as this tends to shallow the upper fornix.

Contracted socket

Congenital small socket

The most extreme form of contracted socket occurs in children born without an eye (anophthalmos) or with a very small eye (microphthalmos). The management is to fit expanders into the socket at as young an age as possible to stretch the tissue and try to stimulate conjunctival, lid, and bony orbital growth. Various expanders can be tried from the conventional fitting of a series of larger shapes to the use of hydrophilic shapes or silicone balloons which can be progressively inflated. These can be placed either within the conjunctival sac or in the orbit itself, which may produce better bone expansion. When no further expansion of the tissues can be achieved with conservative measures, consideration must be given to enlarging the soft tissues with mucous membrane grafts and possible skin flaps and enlarging the bony orbit with bone grafts.

Box 9.3 Causes of contracted socket

Congenital
- Anophthalmos
- Microphthalmos

Acquired
- Radiotherapy
- Alkaline or chemical burns
- Fractured orbit
- Chronic infection especially if associated with extrusion of the implant
- Failure to wear prosthesis
- Excessive loss of conjunctiva during enucleation

Acquired contracted socket

Mild contracture

This may present with an upper or lower lid entropion which can be corrected with entropion surgery.

Localised contracture

A band of contracted mucous membrane may be elongated using a Z-plasty technique.

Severe contracture

If there is severe shortage of socket lining a graft must be used to supplement the deficient conjunctiva. When the socket is moist, buccal mucous membrane is the preferred material. In a dry socket split skin may be employed but the results are often disappointing. If skin is used to line a moist socket it tends to desquamate and may lead to irritation and discharge. If the socket is volume deficient and mildly contracted a dermofat graft can be used to correct both these defects.

In severely contracted sockets or postexenteration sockets a spectacle borne prosthesis may be more acceptable than attempted major surgical reconstruction.

Discharging sockets

Socket discharge is a problem frequently encountered in patients with prostheses.

Causes

Prosthesis

- *Poor fit.* Dead space occurring behind the prosthesis allowing pooling of secretions
- *Mechanical irritation* – Scratched or cracked prosthesis
- *Hypersensitive reaction* to the prosthetic material (methylmethacrylate) or to protein deposited on the surface of the prosthesis
- *Poor prosthesis hygiene.*

Orbital implant

- *Extrusion of the implant.* Partially extruded implant producing irritation and increased secretions

- *Conjunctival inclusion cysts* produced by implantation of conjunctiva or epithelial downgrowth at the site of implant extrusion
- *Granuloma formation.*

Lids

- *Poor closure.* Shortage of skin and/or conjunctiva; implant too large
- *Infected focus.* Blepharitis or meibomianitis.

Socket lining

Attempts at surgical correction using a mixture of skin and mucous membrane can lead to chronically discharging socket.

Lacrimal system

- *Defective tear production.* Resulting in dry socket with crusting of secretions on the surface of the prosthesis
- *Defective tear drainage.* Because of poorly positioned puncta or nasolacrimal blockage
- *Infected focus.* Such as dacryocystitis producing retrograde spread of infection.

All patients wearing prostheses should be advised to handle them as little as possible In acute infection antibiotic drops should be prescribed. In the case of chronic discharge both steroid and antibiotic drops may be effective after the socket has been swabbed and the scraping sent for microbiology and cytology. Regular polishing of the prosthesis and a viscus lubricant, usually polyvinyl alcohol, may help to clear the prosthesis of dried secretions. If the prosthesis is heavily "caked" patients should be advised to wash the prosthesis in a mild household detergent.

If the implant is extruding this should be addressed and conjunctival inclusion cysts or granulomata excised. Lid and socket surgery should be performed to provide adequate closure over the prosthesis. In mild cases of socket contracture entropion correction is often sufficient but if the socket is grossly contracted, a mucous membrane graft may be necessary. Lid surgery, which repositions the puncta improving epiphora, may be necessary but if nasolacrimal or canalicular blockage exists lacrimal drainage surgery may be required.

Further reading

Collin JRO. *Socket surgery. A manual of systemic eye lid surgery.* London: Churchill Livingstone, 1989.

Dutton JJ. Coralline Hydroxyapatite as an ocular implant. *Ophthalmology* 1991; **98**:370–7.

Jones CA, Collin JROC. A classification and review of the causes of discharging sockets. *Trans Ophthal Soc UK* 1983; **103**:351–3.

Jordan DR, Allen L, Ells A *et al.* The use of Vicryl mesh to implant hydroxyapatite implants. *Ophthal Plast Reconstr Surg* 1995; **11**:95–9.

Jordan DR, Gilberg SM, Mawn L, Grahovac SZ. The synthetic Hydroxyapatite implant: a report on 65 patients. *Ophthal Plast Reconstr Surgery* 1998; **14**:250–5.

Kaltreider SA, Jacobs LJ, Hughes MO. Predicting the ideal implant size before enucleation. *Ophthal Plast Reconstr Surg* 1999; **15**:37–43.

Karesch JW, Dresner SC. High density porous polyethylene (Medpor) as a successful anophthalmic socket implant. *Ophthalmology* 1994; **101**:1688–96.

Levine MR, Pou CR, Lash RH. Evisceration: Is sympathetic ophthalmia a concern in the new millennium. *Ophthal Plast Reconstr Surg* 1999; **15**:4–8.

McNab AA. *Orbital Exenteration. Manual of orbital & lachrymal surgery* (2nd Ed.). Oxford: Butterworth Heinemann, 1998.

Nunery WR, Chen WP. Enucleation and evisceration. In: Bosniak S, ed. *Principles and practice of ophthalmic plastic and reconstructive surgery.* London: WB Saunders, 1995.

Perry AC. Advances in enucleation. *Ophthal Plast Reconstr Surg* 1991; 7:173–82.

Shaefer DP. Evaluation and management of the anophthalmic socket and socket reconstruction. Smith's Ophthalmic Plastic and Reconstructive Surgery (2nd Ed.). London: Mosby, 1997.

Smit TJ, Koornneef L, Zonneveld FW, Groet E, Oho AJ. Primary and secondary implants in the anophthalmic orbit: pre-operative and postoperative computer tomographic appearance. *Ophthalmology* 1991; **98**:106–10.

Smith B, Petrelli R. Dermis fat graft as a movable implant within the muscle cone. *Am J Ophthalmol* 1978; **85**:62–6.

Soll DB. The anophthalmic socket. *Ophthalmology* 1982; **89**: 407–23.

Thaller VT. Enucleated volume measurement. *Ophthalmic Plast Reconstr Surg* 1997; **13**:18–20.

Tyers AG, Collin JRO. Orbital implants and post-enucleation socket syndrome. *Trans Ophthalmol Soc UK* 1982: **102**:90–2.

10 Investigation of lacrimal and orbital disease

Timothy J Sullivan

Although many conditions can affect the orbit, the symptoms of orbital disease are relatively limited (Box 10.1) and most diseases are of structural, inflammatory, infectious, vascular, neoplastic or degenerative origin. A thorough history and systematic examination usually provides the astute clinician with a concise differential diagnosis and will guide appropriate further investigation; in particular, the temporal sequence and speed of events is very important in suggesting the likely disease. A general medical history, a history of trauma or prior malignancy, and a family history of systemic diseases (for example, thyroid or other autoimmune diseases) are also very important.

Box 10.1 Main presenting symptoms of orbital disease

- Pain
- Proptosis
- Globe displacement
- Mass
- Periorbital (including lid) changes

- Visual loss
- Diplopia
- Sensory disturbance
- Epiphora
- Exposure symptoms

Assessment of orbital disease

History taking for orbital disease

Pain

Patients should be questioned closely on the nature, intensity, location, radiation and duration of pain: those with thyroid orbitopathy may, for example, have either deep orbital pain, due to increased intraorbital pressure, or ocular surface pain related to exposure keratopathy. Deep-seated, relentless ache may be found in neoplasia, sclerosing inflammation or with some specific inflammatory diseases, such as Wegener's granulomatosis.

Factors that relieve or exacerbate the pain should be sought, the pain of orbital myositis typically being worse with eye movements away from the field of action of affected muscles. Pain worse during straining or with the head dependent suggests the filling and congestion of a distensible venous anomaly or pain of sinus origin.

Proptosis and globe displacement

Whilst some patients may be aware of displacement of the globe, in some only relatives or friends will have noted these symptoms. Old photographs may be helpful in establishing the duration of displacement.

Posteriorly located lesions cause axial proptosis, while anterior lesions tend to displace the globe away from the mass (Figure 10.1a and

10.1b). Enophthalmos may be seen with post-traumatic enlargement of the orbital cavity, orbital venous anomalies, scirrhous tumours (typically breast or bronchial carcinoma) or with hemifacial atrophy (Figure 10.1c).

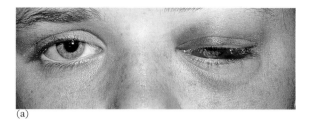

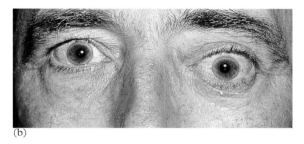
(a)

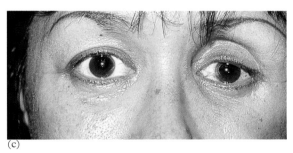
(b)

(c)

Figure 10.1 Various forms of ocular displacement due to orbital disease: (a) axial proptosis associated with intraconal haemorrhage; (b) hypoglobus due to cholesterol granuloma of the frontal bone; (c) enophthalmos due to hemi-facial atrophy.

Variability of globe position is important and proptosis increasing with the Valsalva manoeuvre suggests a distensible venous anomaly. Pulsation may be due to transmission of vascular or cerebro-spinal fluid (CSF) pressure waves. Arterial vascular pulsation is normal in young children, but otherwise occurs with orbital arterio-venous malformations, carotico-cavernous fistulae, or rarely with tumours having a significant arterial supply. CSF pulsation occurs with the sphenoid wing hypoplasia of neurofibromatosis or after surgical removal of the orbital roof.

Visual loss

Sudden loss of vision is often due to a vascular cause and associated nausea and vomiting suggests orbital haemorrhage. Although periorbital or subconjunctival ecchymosis may be evident at presentation, often it does not track forward from the orbit (and become visible) for several days. Vaso-obliterative conditions, such as orbital mucormycosis or Wegener's granulomatosis, may also be associated with multiple cranial nerve deficits.

Optic nerve compression generally causes a progressive loss of function, which the patient will notice as failing colour perception and a "drab", "washed-out" and "grey" quality to their vision. Slow-growing retrobulbar masses may compress the globe and affect vision by inducing hypermetropia (or premature presbyopia) or by causing choroidal folds. Gaze evoked amaurosis – with visual failure on certain ductions – may occur with large and slowly growing retrobulbar masses that stretch the optic nerve.

Diplopia

Double vision arises from neurological deficit, muscle disease or due to distortion of orbital tissues. True binocular diplopia may be intermittent or constant, the images may be displaced horizontally, vertically or obliquely, and the diplopia may be worse in different positions of gaze. Thyroid orbitopathy and trauma are the commonest orbital cause of diplopia, although disease at the apex may cause multiple cranial nerve palsies. Anteriorly located tumours tend to displace the globe rather than cause diplopia.

Sensory disturbance

Although periorbital sensory changes, either paraesthesia or hypaesthesia, are uncommon, they provide a valuable guide to location of orbital disease. Sensory loss may occur with orbital inflammation or with malignant infiltration, particularly perineural spread from orbital or periorbital tumours. Specific enquiry should be made for these symptoms, as most patients will not volunteer them.

Exposure symptoms and epiphora

Where proptosis is associated with lagophthalmos, or an incomplete blink cycle, the patient will often have ocular "grittiness", redness and episodic watering; such symptoms being common, and often very troublesome, in patients with thyroid eye disease.

Examination for orbital disease

To avoid missing important orbital signs, the examination should follow a set sequence: visual functions, ocular displacement, ocular balance and ductions, periorbital functions, intraocular signs and signs of systemic disease.

Visual functions

The best-corrected visual acuity and colour perception should be obtained prior to pupillary examination. Ishihara colour plates, although designed for the assessment of hereditary colour anomalies, provide a widely available test for subtle defects of optic nerve function and the speed of testing and number of errors should be recorded. Likewise, the subjective degree of desaturation of a red target, compared with the normal eye, may be assessed. The pupillary reactions, including an approximate quantitative assessment of a relative afferent pupillary defect, should be tested last.

Evidence of mass

Displacement of the globe in each of the three dimensions should be measured and, if there is a manifest ocular deviation, it is important to assess the position whilst in primary position (if possible), covering the eye not being assessed. Evidence of variation, either with arterial pulsation or with the Valsalva manoeuvre, should be sought and the presence of a palpable thrill or bruit recorded.

The resistance of the globe to retropulsion is hard to assess, but may be markedly increased where intraorbital pressure is raised in thyroid orbitopathy.

The size, shape, texture and fixation of an anterior orbital mass provide guidance to the likely site of origin and possible diagnosis. Tenderness suggests an acute inflammation, such as that seen with dacryoadenitis. Dermoid cysts in the supero-temporal quadrant, when mobile, are typical (Figure 10.2a); when fixed, they may simply have periosteal attachment, or they may extend through a defect in the lateral orbital wall. Fixed lesions in the supero-medial quadrant are usually frontal mucocoeles in adults, but dermoid cysts in children (Figure 10.2b) or – very rarely – an anterior encephalocoele. Soft masses causing swelling of the eyelids should be regarded as infiltrative tumours or inflammation, until otherwise proved, and a "salmon patch" subconjunctival lesion is characteristic of lymphoma (Figure 10.3).

Ocular balance and ductions

Binocular patients should be examined for latent or manifest ocular deviations and the approximate extent of uniocular ductions in the four cardinal positions estimated.

A forced duction (traction) test under topical anaesthesia will assist differentiation of neurological from mechanical causes of restricted eye movements. Likewise, retraction of the globe during an active duction suggests fibrosis of the ipsilateral antagonist muscle, this being a common sign with chronic orbital myositis.

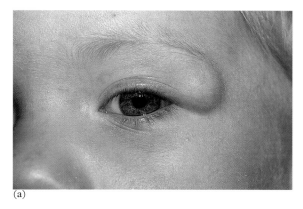

(a)

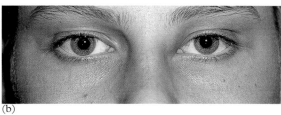

(b)

Figure 10.2   Periocular dermoids: (a) typical lesion in the supero-temporal quadrant; (b) the superomedial dermoid has a differential diagnosis of anterior encephalocoele.

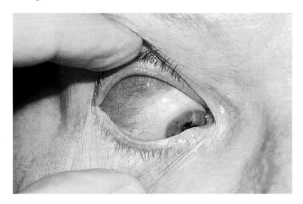

Figure 10.3   Conjunctival "salmon patch" lesion of lymphoma.

Periorbital and eyelid signs

Swelling is the commonest eyelid sign of orbital disease, but lid retraction, lag or incomplete closure are also very common and hallmarks of thyroid orbitopathy (Figure 10.4). An S-shaped contour of the upper lid may be associated with a number of conditions: plexiform neurofibroma of the upper eyelid,

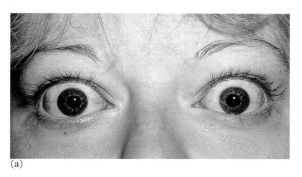

(a)

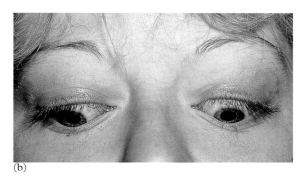

(b)

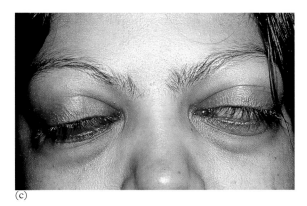

(c)

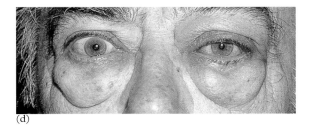

(d)

Figure 10.4   Signs typical of dysthyroid orbitopathy: (a) bilateral proptosis and upper lid retraction; (b) lid lag, best demonstrated by asking the patient to follow a slowly descending target; (c) lagophthalmos on gentle eyelid closure; (d) festoons due to marked periorbital oedema.

101

if present, confirms the diagnosis of peripheral neurofibromatosis; dacryoadenitis, either acute or chronic, may be associated with inflammatory signs; tumours or infiltration of the lacrimal gland. Anterior venous anomalies give a blue hue to eyelid skin and xanthomatous lesions may present as a yellow plaque.

Corkscrew episcleral vessels suggest a low-flow dural shunt (Figure 10.5a) or, in the presence of more extreme vessels and chemosis, a small carotico-cavernous fistula and these are often associated with a raised and widely-swinging intraocular pressure. Markedly dilated, tortuous vessels with a palpable thrill or audible bruit suggest a high-flow carotico-cavernous fistula or arterio-venous malformation (Figure 10.5b). Raised

pressure in the retinal venous circulation leads to loss of the spontaneous pulsation of the central retinal vein, and the presence or absence of pulsation should be noted in both fundi.

Periocular sensory loss should be assessed, as it provides a good guide to location of the orbital disease, and loss of corneal sensation must be noted.

Examination of the nose and mouth is important: palatal varices may indicate orbital varices as a cause of spontaneous orbital haemorrhage, or the presence of a nasal mass or palatal necrosis may indicate a sino-orbital tumour or infection (such as mucormycosis).

Signs of intraocular or systemic disease

Slit lamp bio-microscope examination of the ocular surface and the anterior and posterior segments should be performed: conjunctival chemosis may be seen in inflammatory conditions, including thyroid related ophthalmopathy, and superior limbic kerato-conjunctivitis is typically related to thyroid orbitopathy. The pathognomonic Lisch nodules of neurofibromatosis are readily apparent in the postpubertal patient (Figure 10.6). Anterior or posterior segment inflammation may accompany the orbital inflammatory syndromes as a secondary phenomenon.

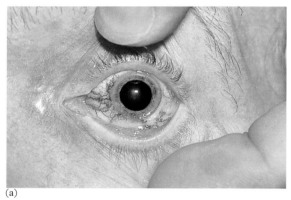

(a)

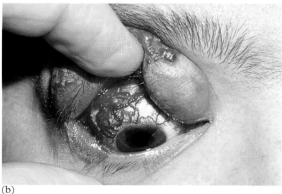

(b)

Figure 10.5 (a) Dilated episcleral veins in a patient with a low-flow dural shunt; (b) the grossly abnormal vasculature, with conjunctival chemosis, in a patient with a high-flow orbital arterio-venous malformation.

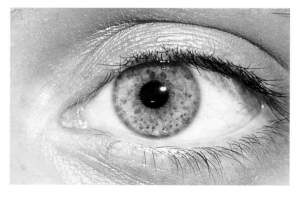

Figure 10.6 Typical Lisch nodules of neurofibromatosis Type I.

With compression of the globe due to tight inferior recti in thyroid orbitopathy, the measured intra-ocular pressure is often elevated during fixation in primary gaze; a true measure of the underlying pressure is given by placing the chin forward, in front of the rest, and having the patient look in slight down-gaze. A widely-swinging pulsation of the mires during applanation tonometry suggests an arterio-venous communication affecting the orbital circulation, or transmitted dural pulsation – as with dysplasia of the sphenoid in neurofibromatosis.

Choroidal striae result from globe indentation by an orbital mass, from optic nerve meningiomas or can be idiopathic; the folds occur almost exclusively at the macula and are not related to the position of the orbital mass. Atrophy or swelling of the optic disc may be due to many causes and optico-ciliary shunt vessels develop with longstanding optic nerve compression as, for example, with optic nerve meningioma.

The regional lymph nodes should be examined for enlargement or tenderness, and the presence of widespread lymphadenopathy sought. Lymphadenopathy, particularly where due to haematological malignancy, may be associated with splenomegaly. In a patient with an orbital mass, clubbing of the finger-nails may indicate underlying bronchogenic carcinoma and the changes of thyroid acropachy or pretibial myxoedema would suggest thyroid orbitopathy.

Ancillary tests in orbital disease

Visual field assessment provides additional information, together with a permanent record, of optic nerve function and may be either static or kinetic tests.

Fields of monocular ductions are somewhat variable, but large changes with time may be of value in monitoring the severity and treatment of thyroid orbitopathy involving the extraocular muscles. Likewise, serial measurement of the field of binocular single vision (BSV) and Hess chart is a useful and permanent record of binocular motility and balance in various orbital conditions, such as thyroid ophthalmopathy, orbital fractures and orbital myositis.

The clinical and imaging features of most orbital conditions will guide the clinician toward the correct diagnosis and for some there may be appropriate systemic blood tests (Table 10.1). Diagnosis of specific forms of inflammatory orbital disease remains elusive.

Table 10.1 Systemic investigations in orbital disease.

Orbital disease	Tests for causative systemic diseases
Thyroid orbitopathy	Ultra-sensitive TSH Free T3, Free T4 TSH receptor antibodies Anti-peroxidase antibodies Anti-thyroglobulin antibodies
Orbital cellulitis	Full blood count Blood cultures (Cultures of abscess contents)
Orbital inflammatory disease	Full blood count Erythrocyte sedimentation rate C-reactive protein Angiotensin converting enzyme Syphilis serology Sputum acid fast bacilli, Mantoux Viral serology (EBV, coxsackie) Bartonella henselae (Cat Scratch disease) cANCA, pANCA Antiproteinase-3 Vascular endothelial growth factor Anti nuclear antibody Anti double stranded DNA Extractable nuclear antigens Rheumatoid factor Ro and La antibodies (Sjogrens)
Orbital haemorrhage	Full blood count (film) Activated partial thromboplastin time Prothrombin time Thrombin time Fibrinogen Factor VIII Ristocetin Platelet desegregation time Bleeding time
Metastasis	Carcinoembryonic antigen Prostate specific antigen Vanillylmandelic acid Homovanillic acid

Orbital ultrasonography

With orbital diseases, ultrasonography is principally of value in examination of the intraocular structure (where ultrasonographic resolution is greater than CT or MRI) and for the examination of vascular size and flow-rates, using colour-coded Doppler ultrasonography. It is, therefore, particularly useful for the detection of small intraocular tumours, intraocular tumours in the presence of opaque media, scleritis and inflammation in the posterior Tenon's space, arterio-venous malformations and low- or high-flow vascular shunts.

With orbital vascular anomalies, there may be not only enlargement of the superior ophthalmic vein (compared with the normal side), but also an arterial wave-form to the flow, together with reversal of direction of flow within the vein.

Computed tomography

As the orbit and surrounding sinuses have tissues with naturally high radiographic contrast, thin-slice computed tomography is the most effective and economical tool for the initial imaging of the orbit (Figure 10.7).

For a suspected orbital mass, a single run of axial scans with intravenous contrast (unless contraindicated), together with coronal reformats images, is generally sufficient to give a probable diagnosis and allow planning of surgery or medical therapy; if needed, direct coronal imaging may give greater detail of the relationship of the mass to the optic nerve or rectus muscles. For planning the repair of blowout fractures, or the diagnosis and treatment of thyroid orbitopathy, a single run of direct coronal scans (without contrast) is often sufficient. Parasagittal reformats along the plane of the vertical recti and optic nerve may also be of help in orbital floor trauma and in evaluating the relationship of lesions to the optic nerve (Figure 10.8).

For orbital pathology arising in bone, or where secondary bone invasion is suspected, then it is important to obtain images with

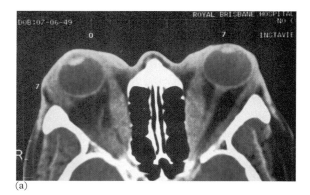

(a)

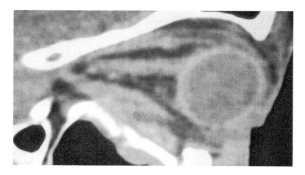

(b)

Figure 10.7　A patient with dysthyroid orbitopathy, showing gross proptosis and enlargement of extraocular muscles, as imaged by (a) axial and (b) coronal soft tissue CT scans through the mid-orbits.

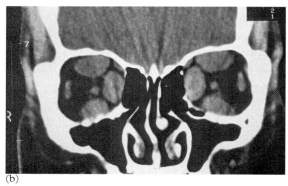

Figure 10.8　Parasagittal reformatted CT, imaged along the line of the vertical recti, showing the inferior rectus muscle to be free from the site of a repaired orbital floor fracture.

both soft tissue and bone window settings. Spiral CT allows greatly reduced imaging time and three-dimensional studies may be of help in planning major cranio-facial reconstruction (Figure 10.9).

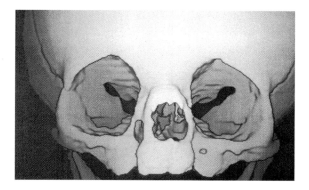

Figure 10.9 Three-dimensional CT reformat for a patient with severe clefting of the facial soft tissues and bone.

Magnetic resonance imaging

Magnetic resonance imaging is derived from the signal emission when hydrogen nuclei realign to a very strong magnetic field after the cessation of an exciting radio frequency pulse, the interval being termed the "relaxation time". Various relaxation times may be assessed and images derived from the measured signals at these different relaxation times: T1-weighted images tend to show anatomical detail of the orbit, whereas T2-weighted images – where the high signal of tissue oedema is readily evident – generally demonstrate pathological processes.

Orbital fat has a high signal on T1-weighting, this often hindering the discernment of orbital pathology, but the contrast can be markedly improved by use of fat-suppression software programmes to manipulate the images. Gadolinium-DTPA provides an intravenous contrast, highlighting vascular lesions or tissues with leaking vessels (Figure 10.10) but with T1-weighted images, renders pathology less discernable unless used in conjunction with fat-suppression.

MRI should not be used routinely for the investigation of orbital disease, but provides additional information to CT in certain circumstances. It is of particular value in determining the nature of optic nerve lesions in the region of the optic canal and chiasm; in demonstrating the position of the optic nerve

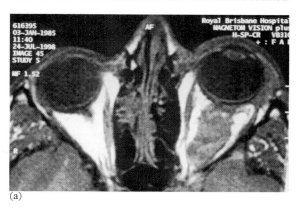

(a)

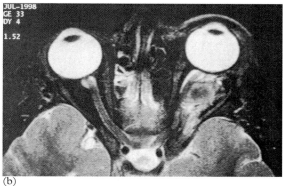

(b)

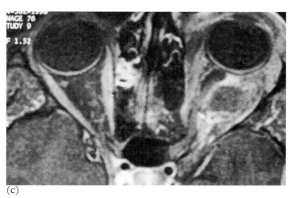

(c)

Figure 10.10 MRI of a patient with recent intraconal orbital haemorrhage: (a) T1- and (b) T2-weighted images, and (c) fat-suppressed T1-weighted image with Gadolinium-DTPA, showing normal uptake of contrast in the extraocular muscles on the unaffected right side. A fluid level may be seen within the lesion of the left orbit.

within large orbital tumours, where not shown on CT; in the imaging of radiolucent foreign bodies that are not ferro-magnetic. Although the presence of muscular oedema on STIR images is suggestive of active inflammatory oedema in patients with thyroid orbitopathy, MRI used for this purpose is expensive and does not add usefully to a thorough clinical examination.

Although there are exceptions, most orbital tumours have a fairly low T1 signal, a medium-to-high T2 signal, and show variable Gadolinium-DTPA enhancement. Non-specific orbital inflammation tends to have a medium T1 signal, with a relatively low signal on T2. Lesions containing melanin, or the breakdown products of blood, and those with lipid, fat or mucus will give high signal on T1-weighted images; examples include orbital haemorrhage, orbital melanomas, cholesterol granulomas, dermoid cysts and sinus mucocoeles.

Angiography

Magnetic resonance angiography offers information on the vascular dynamics of most orbital lesions, although intra-arterial contrast angiography (selective internal and external carotid arteriography) remains important in the exclusion of small aneurysms, dural low flow arterio-venous fistulae and the investigation of pulsatile proptosis not explained by other imaging modalities. Another important indication is in the surgical planning of high flow tumours, such as haemangiopericytoma, and consideration of therapeutic embolisation of the arterial supply may be considered at the time of angiography.

Positron emission tomography (PET) and single photon emission CT (SPECT)

These modalities have yet to find a major place in orbital assessment, but may become important in the coming decade. Current uses include staging patients with non-small cell carcinoma of the lung, malignant melanoma, Hodgkin's disease, non-Hodgkin's lymphoma, colorectal carcinoma and head and neck carcinoma.

PET scanning using fluorine-labelled deoxyglucose radiotracer has proved as reliable as conventional scanning for the identification of primary or metastatic tumour and is also superior to clinical examination or other imaging modalities for detecting nodal metastases; unfortunately the imaging technique presently lacks anatomic detail. A major current role, particularly in patients with lymphoma, is in the differentiation of tumour from fibrous tissue after radiotherapy.

Octreotide scintigraphy

Following the discovery of somatostatin receptors on the activated lymphocytes associated with thyroid orbitopathy, radio-labelled octreotide (a somatostatin analogue) has been used as a semi-objective tool in the evaluation of the disease activity in this condition. The test is extremely expensive and its use limited to a few research centres.

Tissue diagnosis

Tissue diagnosis remains essential for the appropriate management of almost every orbital disease. Although fine needle aspiration biopsy is useful for the confirmation of certain tumours in a patient with known systemic malignancy, it requires an experienced cytologist to interpret results. Even with CT or ultrasonographic guidance, fine-needle aspiration of post-equatorial lesions is hazardous and the amount of tissue often insufficient for the histological studies required. Most experienced orbital surgeons favour an open biopsy approach, in order to correctly identify pathological tissue, secure haemostasis, and obtain enough tissue for pathological studies.

Assessment of lacrimal drainage disease

The patient presenting with a watering eye may be producing too many tears, may have trouble delivering the tears to the drainage apparatus, or may have defective tear drainage. Hypersecretion is usually due to ocular surface irritation, trichiasis, or blepharitis. The lacrimal pump relies on intact motor nerve supply from the facial nerve, good tone in the orbicularis oculi muscle and taut lids to deliver tears to the lacrimal drainage apparatus. The drainage apparatus can be intrinsically affected at the level of the puncti, canaliculi, lacrimal sac and the nasolacrimal duct, and can also be adversely affected by nasal pathology. A thorough history and meticulous examination will usually aid the elucidation of this polyfactorial symptom.

History for patients with lacrimal disease

Apart from helping to elucidate the cause of the epiphora, the history (Box 10.2) allows assessment of the degree of functional disturbance to the patient. In some, epiphora is simply a mild nuisance, whereas in others it significantly interferes with their quality of life, often with a profound effect on reading and driving. In most cases tears spill over at the medial canthus, whereas lateral spillover usually occurs with lower lid laxity (Figure 10.11). The nature of the discharge, whether water, mucus, pus or blood-stained tears, is a useful guide to the likely type of block; blood-stained tears, although most commonly due to severe Actinomyces canaliculitis, may indicate a tumour of the lacrimal drainage system. Bilateral epiphora associated with itching, foreign body sensation, pain or photophobia is indicative of reflex hypersecretion. Obstructive epiphora is often unilateral and usually worse outdoors in cold, windy conditions. A history of cicatrising conditions such as trachoma, herpes simplex, Stevens-Johnson syndrome, systemic chemotherapy with 5-fluorouracil, ocular chemical burns or chronic ocular medication, and pemphigoid should raise suspicion of canalicular disease.

> **Box 10.2 Main aspects of history from the lacrimal patient**
>
> - Duration of symptoms
> - Unilateral or bilateral
> - Severity
> - Constant or intermittent
> - Precipitating factors (for example, cold or windy weather)
> - Spillover of tears at medial or lateral canthus
> - Associated symptoms (for example, discharge, blurred vision, skin excoriation)
> - Past history: cicatricial skin or ocular diseases, herpetic disease, eyelid trauma, dacryocystitis
> - Chronic nasal disease, nasal injury and surgery to the nose or sinuses
> - Drug history: including topical medications, anticoagulants, antiplatelet drugs
> - Fitness for surgery

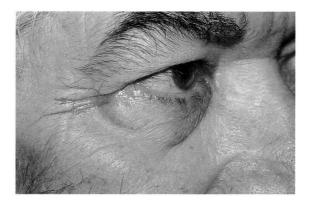

Figure 10.11 Lateral canthal spillover of dye in a patient with lower lid laxity as the main cause for epiphora.

Examination of patients with lacrimal disease

Careful examination of the eyelids and ocular surface should exclude causes of hypersecretion such as marginal blepharitis (Figure 10.12),

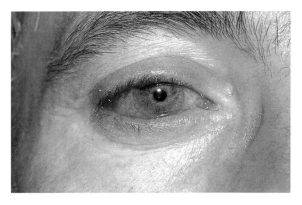

Figure 10.12   Epiphora caused by severe blepharo-keratitis in a patient with acne rosacea.

trichiasis, dry eyes, pingueculum and corneal pathology.

The normal punctum is directed into the tear lake and, although frank lower lid ectropion is easily recognisable, mild punctal ectropion may be missed and is often associated with secondary punctal stenosis. A pouting punctum with a plug of stringy pus that is almost impossible to express is suggestive of Actinomyces canaliculitis (Figure 10.13). Eyelid laxity, even in the absence of lid or punctal malposition, can result in troublesome epiphora due to lacrimal pump failure and "gravitation" of the tear-line on the sagging lower lid margin. Facial weakness should be noted and the presence of aberrant

muscular movements suggests aberrant reinnervation and the possibility of "crocodile tears" as a cause of the patient's symptoms. The presence of a lacrimal sac mucocoele or a mass may only become evident after palpation of the lacrimal sac fossa; a readily expressible mucocoele suggests a patent canalicular system with nasolacrimal duct obstruction and requires no further investigation.

Each tear film should be stained with a partial drop of 2% fluorescein and the height of the tear meniscus and stability (break-up time) of the tear film assessed. Corneal staining suggests the possibility of episodic reflex hypersecretion due to unstable tear film or reduced background tear secretion. The rate of dye disappearance from the conjunctival sac, particularly useful in children, gives a good indication of lacrimal drainage especially when both sides are compared (Figure 10.14).

Lacrimal syringing is invariably performed as part of the assessment of the adult patient with epiphora. Good technique is essential not only to obtain maximum information, but also to avoid canalicular damage and subsequent fibrosis; it is possible that many canalicular obstructions are iatrogenic. After instilling a topical anaesthetic, the punctum may be dilated without rupturing the surrounding ring of connective tissue or annulus. Lateral traction is applied to the eyelid to straighten the canaliculus and a fine lacrimal cannula on a 2ml saline-filled syringe is used to gently probe the appropriate canaliculus (Figure 10.15). In cases of canalicular obstruction a

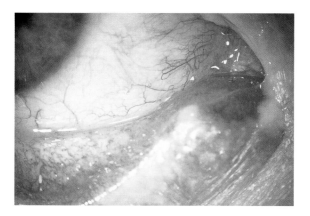

Figure 10.13   Stringy, non-expressible pus at the punctum of a canaliculus affected by Actinomyces.

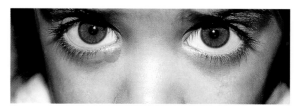

Figure 10.14   Asymmetrical tear lines and dye disappearance in a child with nasolacrimal duct stenosis.

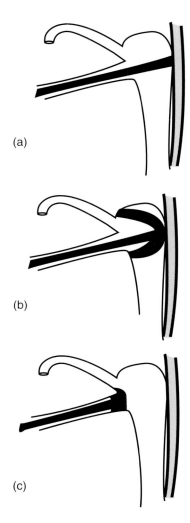

(a)

(b)

(c)

Figure 10.15 Analysis of lacrimal probing and syringing: (a) "hard stop" with a patent canalicular system; (b) medial "soft stop" with obstruction of common canaliculus; (c) lateral "soft stop" due to lower canalicular obstruction.

lacrimal sac and, in such cases, the irrigation fluid that reaches the nose if the nasolacrimal duct is patent or only partially obstructed; reflux of fluorescein-stained fluid, with or without mucus, from opposite punctum and failure of fluid to reach the nose indicates total nasolacrimal duct obstruction.

Intranasal examination (with a headlight and speculum or, ideally, an endoscope) may be performed, looking for the presence of fluorescein in the inferior meatus, polyps, allergic rhinitis, septal deviation, turbinate impaction (rare), or other intranasal diseases (Figure 10.16). Preoperative nasal endoscopy is essential in the assessment of patients for endonasal lacrimal procedures.

Ancillary tests for lacrimal assessment

Dacryocystography

Dacryocystography provides very good anatomical detail of the outflow system – revealing occlusion, stenosis or dilatation of the outflow tract and also, in some cases, diverticulae, stones, or tumour (Figure 10.17) – but does not give a true measure of the physiological function. However, where the system is patent during injection of contrast, the failure of spontaneous clearance of oil-based contrast media after the patient resumes

"soft stop" is reached. Reflux of *clear* fluid through the same punctum in individual canalicular obstruction or through the opposite punctum in common canalicular obstruction: with individual canalicular obstruction, the point of obstruction may be assessed by grasping the cannula at the punctum with fine forceps before withdrawing it from the canaliculus. In the absence of canalicular disease a "hard stop" is felt as the cannula reaches the medial wall of the

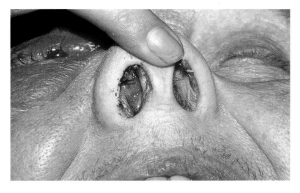

Figure 10.16 Intranasal tumour causing epiphora.

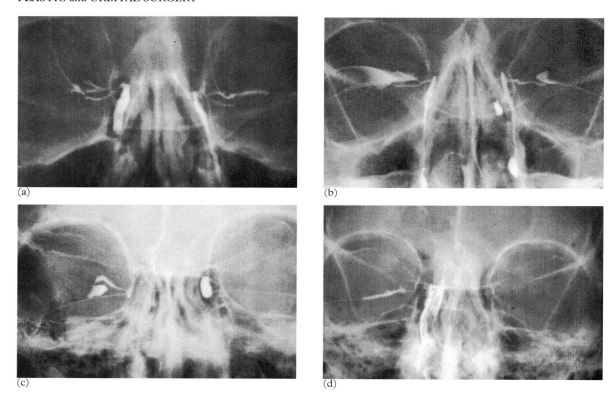

Figure 10.17 Dacryocystography showing: (a) an anatomically normal left system but a dilated right lacrimal sac with filling defect due to a stone; (b) an anatomically normal right system (although contrast reflux suggests distal stenosis within the outflow tract) and a tiny, non-functional left surgical anastomosis after endonasal dacryocystorhinostomy, (c) a small right and large left mucocoele; (d) a functional right dacryocystorhinostomy with direct drainage of contrast to the nasal space.

the upright posture is suggestive of a reduced physiological clearance (so-called "functional block").

Dacryocystography is indicated in planning endonasal lacrimal surgery, or with surgery for congenital lacrimal anomalies, after trauma, after cranio-facial repair, with revisional lacrimal surgery, or where a tumour or sequestrum within the system is suspected. A dilated canalicular system with filling defects may be evident in Actinomyces canaliculitis (Figure 10.18). There is no indication for dacryocystography where clinical signs indicate an uncomplicated lacrimal sac mucocoele.

Lacrimal drainage scintigraphy

This study uses a gamma camera to follow the passage of a drop of radio-labelled fluid

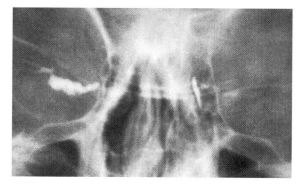

Figure 10.18 A typically dilated canaliculus in a patient with Actinomyces canaliculitis.

(usually Technetium 99) from the conjunctival sac to the nasal passages, and provides a measure of physiological tear clearance where there is a patent system on clinical

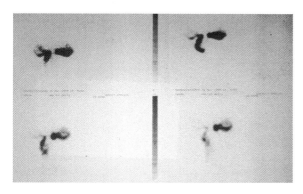

Figure 10.19 Lacrimal scintigraphy showing a normal right drainage pattern but a marked delay in the exit of tracer from the left lacrimal sac.

examination or dacryocystography (Figure 10.19). In this situation, scintigraphy will generally reveal whether there is a failure of gathering of tears into the drainage system (often due to lid anomalies), or a failure of clearance of tears that are otherwise rapidly entering the system from the tear lake.

Computed tomography

Computed tomography is indicated when a lacrimal sac tumour is suspected and may be helpful in planning surgery for trauma cases, particularly when plating systems have been used. Craniofacial disorders and sclerosing bony dysplasias may have unusual bone anatomy shown on CT, and these changes may influence the approach to surgery and the prognosis.

11 Dysthyroid eye disease

Carol Lane

Dysthyroid eye disease is the commonest cause of proptosis in adults and the disease typically presents as Graves' disease in the third and fourth decade, with a four- to seven-fold predominance in females. Bilateral orbital inflammation is often accompanied by eyelid retraction and restriction of ocular movements. Asymmetrical involvement and extensive fibrosis are less frequent presentations and the diagnosis of dysthyroid eye disease should always be suspected in the presence of any inflamed orbit or with proptosis.

Sight is threatened by corneal exposure due to incomplete eyelid closure over a proptotic globe, uncontrolled ocular hypertension or optic nerve compression. One-fifth of patients with untreated compressive optic neuropathy develop irreversible visual impairment (to 6/36 or less).

Treatment of dysthyroid eye disease aims to conserve or restore normal visual function, relieve ocular pain and achieve an acceptable appearance.

Pathogenesis

In Graves' hyperthyroidism it is likely that thyroid damage leads to activation of autoimmune thyroid disease by activation of anti-receptor antibodies to the thyrotrophin receptor (TSH receptor). Eye disease is clinically evident in 40% of patients with Graves' disease but, in contrast, in only 3% of patients with Hashimoto's thyroiditis and very rarely with primary hypothyroidism. The high correlation between Graves' disease and orbital disease suggests a shared antigen, such as TSH receptor, thyroglobulin or thyroid peroxidase. Circulating activated T lymphocytes infiltrate the orbital tissues, where they release cytokines which, in turn, stimulate proliferation of fibroblasts and deposition of glycosaminoglycans (GAGs). Intense lymphocytic infiltration, fibroblast proliferation and perimysial oedema result in expansion of orbital contents and proptosis. Subsequent fibrosis of involved perimysial connective tissue results in varying degrees of muscular contracture.

Hales and Rundle described the natural history of dysthyroid eye disease, with the disease typically peaking after six months and active inflammation resolving within 18 months. Of 67 patients followed for an average of 15 years, those with gross eye disease persisting for more than six months after control of thyroid status had a worse outcome. The disease tends to be more severe in males and in smokers, and the elongated myopic globe is at greater risk of exposure keratopathy, whereas a tight orbit without proptosis is at greater risk of compressive optic neuropathy (Figure 11.1).

Features of dysthyroid eye disease

Although Werner's early "NOSPECS" classification of dysthyroid eye disease

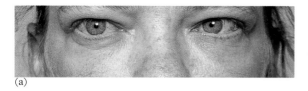

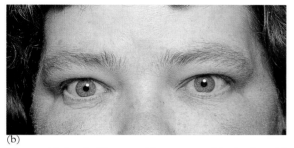

Figure 11.1 A 39-year-old woman with dysthyroid compressive optic neuropathy: (a) before and (b) after orbital decompression.

Table 11.1 Assessment of common clinical features of dysthyroid eye disease (after *Thyroid* 1992; 2:235–6).

Feature	Clinical assessment
Eyelid	Maximal fissure width Upper lid to limbus distance and lower lid to limbus distance
Cornea	Exposure keratopathy assessed by Rose Bengal or fluorescein staining (indicates presence of absence of staining)
Extraocular muscles	Binocular single vision in central 30° field (indicate presence or absence, with or without prisms) and one or more of the following measurement techniques: Maddox rod test; alternate cover test; Hess chart or Lancaster red–green test. Optional: intraocular pressures, CT scan or MRI scan
Proptosis	Exophthalmometry (CT or MRI scan may also be used for measurement)
Optic nerve activity score	Visual acuity, fields and colour vision Sum one point for each of the following: spontaneous retrobulbar pain; pain with eye movement; eyelid erythema; eyelid oedema; conjunctival injection; conjunctival chemosis; caruncular swelling
Patient self-assessment	Satisfaction with the following (indicate change of each with therapy, using a scale such as "greatly improved, improved, unchanged, worse, much worse"): appearance; subjective visual function; ocular discomfort; diplopia

underlines the concept of a gradation of severity of the condition, it has largely been superseded by classifications based upon the degree of inflammation – such as that of Mourits or that of others (Table 11.1). A simple "activity score" may be assigned by awarding one point for each of retrobulbar pain, pain on eye movement, eyelid erythema, eyelid oedema, conjunctival injection, conjunctival chemosis, caruncular swelling, deteriorating vision, diplopia and worsening appearance; an activity score of 3 or more (out of 10) indicates active disease.

An objective deterioration in visual acuity, reduced colour perception, an acquired visual field defect, impaired visual-evoked potentials or corneal ulceration are signs of serious sight-threatening disease for which urgent intervention is essential.

Treatment of the thyrotoxicosis of Graves' disease tends to improve eye signs, although hypothyroidism after suppression of the hyperthyroid state may exacerbate ophthalmopathy and this should be avoided by regular blood tests during control of the thyroid gland. Recent evidence suggests that radio-iodine treatment for thyrotoxicosis may adversely affect ophthalmopathy and systemic steroids during therapy may prevent exacerbation of the eye disease.

Although most patients with the clinical features of dysthyroid eye disease have abnormal thyroid function, some will be euthyroid and the clinical diagnosis may be supported only by raised levels of serum thyroid auto-antibodies.

Orbital imaging in dysthyroid eye disease (most readily with CT scan) tends to show enlargement of several extraocular muscles, the inferior and medial recti being affected most frequently, the superior and lateral recti less often and involvement of the oblique muscles being relatively rare. Other features include changes in the orbital fat and, with longstanding disease, changes in the thin

Box 11.1 Typical features of dysthyroid eye disease on CT or MR imaging

- Enlarged extraocular muscles; tendinous insertion often spared
- Orbital fat normal, diffusely increased opacity or increased in quantity
- Occasional slight bowing of the medial orbital wall (lamina papyracea); the "Coca-Cola bottle" sign
- Frequent inferior rectus enlargement on axial scan, the mass of which may simulate an orbital tumour
- Crowding of the optic nerve, at the orbital apex, by enlarged extraocular muscles
- Lacrimal gland rarely enlarged, but often prolapsed forwards
- Fat prolapse from the orbit into the cranium at the superior orbital fissure
- Absence of orbital masses, vascular anomaly or sinus involvement

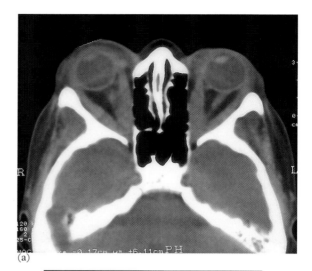

(a)

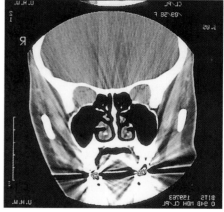

(b)

Figure 11.2 (a) Axial and (b) coronal CT for a patient with compressive optic neuropathy, shown in Figure 11.1. All extraocular muscles are enlarged and there is loss of the fat planes around the optic nerve at the orbital apex.

orbital walls (Box 11.1). Enlargement of the posterior part of the medial rectus is most likely to crowd the orbital apex and cause optic neuropathy (Figure 11.2a) and direct coronal CT scans are valuable for showing "crowding" of the optic nerve at the orbital apex, with loss of the fat spaces, in compressive optic neuropathy (Figure 11.2b). MRI scans, particularly STIR (short-tau inversion recovery) sequences, may provide an indication of the water content of extraocular muscles – this being a reflection of the degree of inflammatory myositis – but the relatively costly investigation adds little to clinical examination. Likewise, B-mode ultrasonography may be used to assess the size of the anterior part of the extraocular muscles, but provides poor images of the posterior orbital structure.

Treatment of dysthyroid eye disease

Most patients with thyroid eye disease will have relatively few symptoms and signs, and many will require only topical lubricants during the active phase of the disease and no long-term therapy. Patients without proptosis when the disease is inactive, but with persistent lid retraction or incomplete lid closure, may need eyelid surgery to protect the cornea (Chapter 7). Likewise, squint surgery may be needed when the eye disease has been shown to be stable and inactive for some months.

Management of more severe and significant thyroid eye disease should be first directed towards suppression of orbital inflammation and later the restoration of orbital function.

Suppression of orbital inflammation in dysthyroid eye disease

Patients with significant signs or symptoms of active orbital inflammation, or with optic neuropathy or significant exposure keratopathy, should receive systemic therapy to reduce the degree of orbital inflammatory congestion. Those with an activity score of 3 or more are likely to benefit, as are those with a muscle oedema shown on STIR-sequence MRI.

Systemic steroids at high dosage (either intravenous methyl prednisolone or oral prednisolone) should be administered and the patient checked for improvement after a few days. The patient should be monitored for hyperglycaemia and hypertension during treatment and the prescription of a gastric proton-pump inhibitor or Histamine-2 receptor antagonist considered; patients on long-term steroids, especially the elderly, should be given calcium supplementation to counteract steroid-induced osteoporosis. If systemic steroids produce an improvement in the inflammatory orbitopathy, the dosage should be slowly reduced towards about 20mg daily if possible and the patient referred for low-dose, (2000–2400 cGy) lens-sparing radiotherapy to the posterior tissues of the orbit; some authors consider radiotherapy contraindicated in diabetics, as it may hasten the development of retinopathy.

Steroids probably suppress dysthyroid orbitopathy by inhibition of the production of cytokines by activated T cells and macrophages and fibroblasts within the orbit. It has been reported that treatment with steroids and radiotherapy is more effective than treatment of orbitopathy with steroids alone. As there may be an increase in orbital inflammation and oedema whilst undergoing orbital radiotherapy, it is prudent to continue a moderate steroid dosage (for example, prednisolone 20mg daily) during this treatment.

Surgical rehabilitation of the patient with dysthyroid eye disease

Severe conjunctival chemosis is self-perpetuating due to the "throttling" effect of the lower eyelid on the prolapsed conjunctiva and will, in some patients, prevent eyelid closure (Figure 11.3a). After subconjunctival injection of local anaesthetic with adrenaline, drainage of subconjunctival fluid and placement of Frost sutures in the upper and lower eyelids will typically allow closure of the eyelids under an occlusive dressing, with topical application of a steroidal ointment (Figure 11.3b). This typically produces a dramatic improvement within 12 hours (Figure 11.3c), allows the cornea to rehydrate and gives time for systemic antiinflammatory therapy to act.

Orbital decompression is necessary if visual function deteriorates despite the use of high-dose systemic steroids (Figure 11.1b). As compression of the optic nerve occurs mainly at the orbital apex, decompression for visual failure must include removal of the posterior part of the medial wall (Figure 11.4); in a few patients the most posterior part of the medial wall being the lateral wall of the sphenoid sinus. Pre-operative CT is required to confirm the diagnosis (especially with unilateral disease), to exclude underlying sinus disease and to detect any cranio-facial anomalies, such as a midline encephalocoele.

Although Olivari has described reduction of proptosis by meticulous excision of orbital fat from the intraconal and extraconal spaces, most orbital decompressions involve removal

115

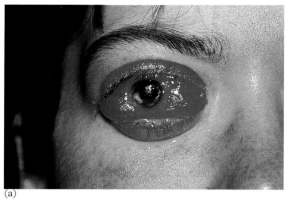

(a)

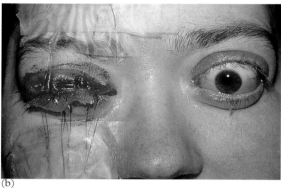

(b)

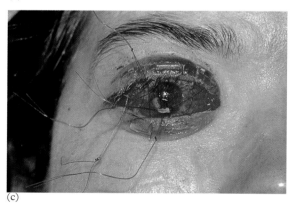

(c)

Figure 11.3 (a) Severe conjunctival chemosis preventing any movement of the right eyelid and causing dehydration of the right cornea. After drainage of the chemosis under local anaesthesia and placement of multiple eyelid traction sutures (b), the eyelid was padded closed for 12 hours with a dramatic improvement in the clinical state (c).

of a combination of the medial wall, floor and lateral wall of the orbit. Removal of the medial wall is necessary for relief of optic neuropathy (Figure 11.5), removal of the floor adds the

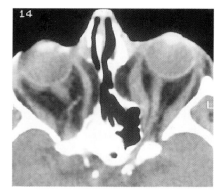

(a)

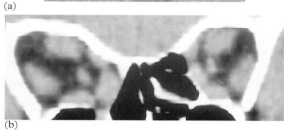

(b)

Figure 11.4 Patient referred with persistent compressive optic neuropathy on the left side, due to the failure to remove the posterior half of the left medial orbital wall. The right side had successful relief of optic neuropathy after a complete ethmoidectomy reaching the orbital apex.

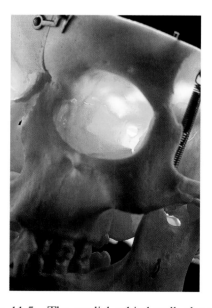

Figure 11.5 The medial orbital wall, showing the lamina papyracea with the foramina for the anterior and posterior ethmoidal arteries in relation to the optic canal.

most to reduction in proptosis and removal of the lateral wall allows reduction of lacrimal gland prolapse and reduces the deleterious effect of medial wall decompression on ocular muscle balance. Decompression requires adequate hypotensive general anaesthesia and a reverse Trendelenburg positioning of the patient to reduce bleeding during this complex surgery.

Other surgery for dysthyroid eye disease

Upper eyelid retraction in thyroid eye disease occurs due to a combination of primary factors (adrenergic stimulation, inflammation and fibrosis) and secondary retraction due to inferior rectus fibrosis – with secondary overaction of the superior rectus/levator complex. If secondary upper eyelid retraction is present, the restriction of ocular motility should be addressed first, with inferior rectus recession. Primary upper eyelid retraction is treated by one of the several techniques for graded levator tenotomy (Chapter 7), but with all methods it is particularly important to completely divide the lateral horn of the levator aponeurosis and to maintain a levator action on the medial part of the upper eyelid.

Lower lid displacement, with excessive scleral show below the lower limbus, is due to proptosis and is almost always corrected by adequate orbital decompression – which should probably be considered in any patient with exophthalmos of 24 mm or more. True lower lid *retraction,* due to an overaction of the retractor fascia in the lower lid, probably occurs only after inferior rectus recession. Lower lid retraction may require surgery to elevate the eyelid using an implant of sclera, hard palate mucosa or ear cartilage.

Lateral tarsorrhaphy invariably stretches with time and, with appropriate surgery to address the other position of the globe and upper eyelid, there is almost no indication for this rather disfiguring procedure in the patient with dysthyroid eye disease. Likewise,

skin-reduction blepharoplasty should be used with caution, as removal of anterior lamella in these patients may risk exacerbation of exposure keratopathy.

Methods for bone-removing orbital decompression

Orbital decompression can be achieved through several approaches: transnasal or transantral endoscopic decompression leaves no external incision, but can provide only a limited decompression (of the medial wall and medial part of the floor); likewise, the post-caruncular transconjunctival incision also provides access for medial wall decompression, but can present some surgical difficulty due to the presence of unrestrained orbital fat in the operative field. The lateral canthotomy approach provides the most aesthetic approach for decompression of up to three walls, which may be required where exophthalmos is greater than 25 mm (Figure 11.6).

Although the use of a bicoronal flap for orbital decompression has been widely reported in the past, there is no advantage to the use of this large-incision approach. Likewise, the Lynch incision of the external ethmoidectomy approach often leaves an unsightly scar and gives only limited access – to the medial wall and medial part of the orbital floor.

Lynch external ethmoidectomy approach

A gently curving incision is placed from the medial end of the brow, past the attachment of the medial canthal tendon, towards the orbital floor (Figure 11.7). After securing haemostasis within the orbicularis muscle, the periosteum is opened in front of the anterior lacrimal crest and the lacrimal sac and medial orbital periosteum raised from the bone. The anterior ethmoidal artery may be exposed, cauterised and divided, although this should not be necessary as the artery provides a key landmark to the level of the cribriform plate – the upper limit of decompression.

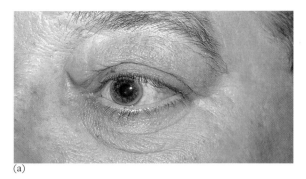

(a)

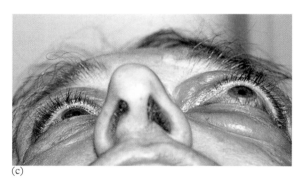

(b)

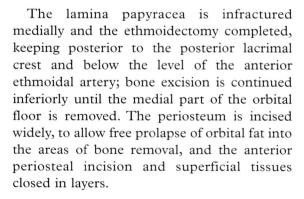

(c)

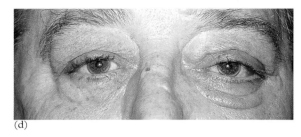

(d)

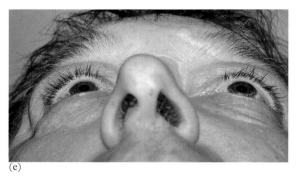

(e)

Figure 11.6 Ten millimetre reduction in left proptosis after three-wall orbital decompression performed through an extended lateral canthotomy incision (a). Preoperative views (b,c) and five weeks after surgery (d,e).

The lamina papyracea is infractured medially and the ethmoidectomy completed, keeping posterior to the posterior lacrimal crest and below the level of the anterior ethmoidal artery; bone excision is continued inferiorly until the medial part of the orbital floor is removed. The periosteum is incised widely, to allow free prolapse of orbital fat into the areas of bone removal, and the anterior periosteal incision and superficial tissues closed in layers.

Extended lateral canthotomy approach

The lateral canthotomy approach (Figure 11.7), with extension of the incision along the lower conjunctival fornix (the "lower lid swinging flap"), provides excellent access to the orbital floor, although decompression of the medial wall requires greater dexterity than with the Lynch approach as access is more restricted. A 1–2 cm extension of the canthotomy into the lateral part of the upper eyelid skin crease (Figure 11.8a) eases access to, and decompression of, the lateral wall.

A horizontal canthotomy of 1.5 cm is made and the orbicularis oculi cauterised and divided infero-laterally to the orbital rim; division of this muscle must be continued until there is a clear release of the lateral tethering of the lower eyelid. The conjunctiva is divided at a point 1 mm below the lower border of the lower tarsus and the conjunctival edge attached to the upper eyelid with a

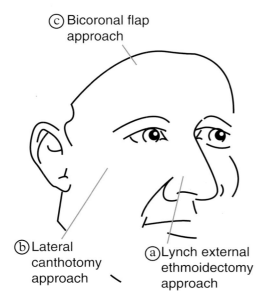

© Bicoronal flap approach

ⓑ Lateral canthotomy approach

ⓐ Lynch external ethmoidectomy approach

Figure 11.7 Incisions for orbital decompression through (a) Lynch external ethmoidectomy approach; (b) lateral canthotomy approach; (c) the bicoronal flap approach.

4/0 nylon suture – this acting to protect the cornea and to keep the lower orbital septum tight during subsequent preparation of a pre-septal skin-muscle flap (Figure 11.8b). The periosteum is opened at the rim, raised widely across the orbital floor and medially up to the level of the ethmoido-frontal suture. The medial part of the orbital floor is fractured with a surgical clip, as much as necessary of the floor and medial wall removed (Figure 11.8c) and the periosteum excised or incised widely over the area of bone removal; it is prudent to preserve the infero-medial bone strut between the maxilla and ethmoid, as this maintains aeration of the maxillary sinus.

If the lateral wall is to be removed, the outer quarter of the upper eyelid skin-crease is divided to reach the level of the superficial temporalis fascia and the periosteum divided 8 mm outside the rim. The periosteum is raised over the rim and into the orbit, the lateral wall removed in part (Figure 11.8d) or whole, and the periosteum below the orbital

lobe of the lacrimal gland incised or excised. The periosteal incision may be continued upwards *just* anterior to the orbital lobe and, when clear of the gland, directed posteriorly along the orbital roof to allow the orbital lobe to fall posteriorly into the defect in the lateral wall (Figure 11.8e) – this repositioning of the gland, together with the marked reduction in proptosis, restoring the depth of the upper eyelid sulcus.

The lateral periosteal strip, to which the intact upper limb of the lateral canthal tendon is still attached, is fixed around the residual bone of the rim and, after placement of a vacuum drain in the intraconal space and sub-temporalis space, the lower fornix incision and canthotomy closed in layers with absorbable sutures.

After instillation of an antibiotic ointment into the conjunctival sac, a 4/0 lower lid traction ("Frost") suture is placed on traction to the forehead and a firm eye dressing applied for 12–18 hours. The vacuum drain and patient are monitored for abnormal haemorrhage.

Subciliary blepharoplasty approach

This approach is similar to the extended lateral canthotomy, except that the preseptal, post-orbicularis plane is reached through a subciliary incision. The technique and view is otherwise identical for the two procedures.

Bicoronal scalp-flap approach

The scalp is shaved 2–3 cm behind the hairline, the operative field prepared and both eyelids closed with tarsorrhaphy sutures. A scalp incision, down to the periosteum, is placed parallel to the hair line (Figure 11.7), compressive haemostatic clips placed, and the flap raised down to the brow ridge. The deep layer of the temporalis fascia is followed down to the level of the zygomatic arch, thereby avoiding branches of the facial nerve.

The pericranium is incised 2 cm above the orbital rim and the periosteal flap raised inferiorly, using (if necessary) an osteotome to

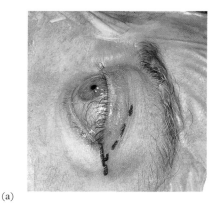

(a)

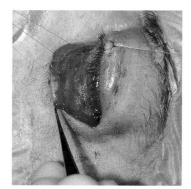

(b)

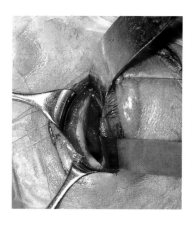

(c)

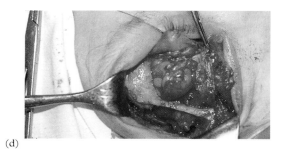

(d)

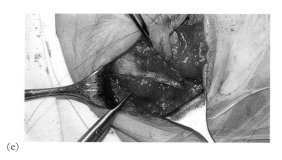

(e)

Figure 11.8   Extended lateral canthotomy approach to orbital decompression: (a) skin incisions for three wall decompression; (b) lower conjunctiva closed over the cornea, with preparation of a lower eyelid swinging flap which provides excellent access to the orbital floor; (c) infraorbital nerve visible after removal of the bone of the orbital floor; (d) the lateral wall has been removed behind an undisturbed orbital rim; (e) the lacrimal gland settles backwards behind the orbital rim, restoring the depth of the upper eyelid sulcus.

release the supraorbital neurovascular bundle from its canal. Using malleable retractors in a hand-over-hand technique, the periosteum is raised across the roof and lateral wall of the orbit and, likewise, the temporalis muscle is raised from its fossa. The thinnest part of the lateral wall is shown by transillumination and an osteotome used to breach the wall at this point, the orbital contents being protected at all times; the breach is extended with rongeurs until adequate lateral wall removal has been accomplished. A series of incisions, to the depth of Richter's muscle, are made in the periosteum above the orbital rim, this increasing flap mobility and reducing thyroid "frown". The medial wall and accessible parts of the orbital floor are removed, the periosteum incised to maximise prolapse of orbital fat and the temporalis fascia closed with 3/0 non-absorbable sutures. Vacuum drains are placed across the subgaleal space from each temporalis fossa, the periosteum closed with a 4/0 absorbable suture and the scalp incision closed with surgical staples. A firm scalp dressing is applied and the vacuum drains maintained until dry.

Post operative management and complications

The patient should be nursed half-seated on bed-rest, to minimise post operative swelling, and (where accessible) the pupils checked for a few hours after surgery. If the patient complains of severe or increasing pain, the affected side should be examined for signs of rising intraorbital pressure due to haemorrhage and appropriate measures taken if it is impairing optic nerve function.

Post operative antibiotics and anti-inflammatory drugs (such as prednisolone 80mg daily, tailing over about ten days) should be administered and the patient instructed to avoid nose-blowing and strenuous exercise over this period. Forced ocular ductions are to be encouraged, as this probably encourages clearance of post operative oedema and recovery of normal ocular balance and movements.

With administration of post operative systemic antibiotics, early infection is rare but sinusitis, particularly maxillary, can be a recurrent late complication of decompression and may require middle meatal antrostomy or other corrective procedure. Under- or over-correction of the proptosis may occur (Figure 11.9a) and, very rarely, the latter (enophthalmos) may be accompanied by hypoglobus.

Loss of vision is extremely rare, but the patient must be made aware of this remote possibility prior to surgery.

Diplopia is almost universal after surgery, will settle within a few weeks in most cases, but presents the greatest practical problems with the activities of daily living. If diplopia is troublesome, it is worthwhile occluding one eye in the early post operative period for those activities (such as descending stairs) where a second image is distracting or dangerous. Where there is no risk with diplopia – as, for example, with watching television – the patient should be encouraged to try and fuse the two images.

Other complications, such as persistent infraorbital neuropraxia, nasolacrimal duct obstruction with epiphora, or secondary lower lid entropion, are uncommon. Likewise, major intraoperative or post operative (Figure 11.9b) haemorrhage, or loss of cerebro-spinal fluid is relatively rare.

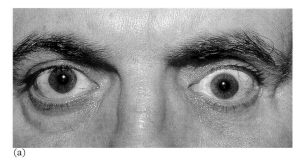
(a)

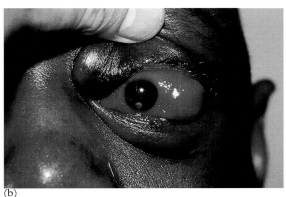
(b)

Figure 11.9   Complications of orbital decompression: (a) late enophthalmos due to maxillary atelectasis; (b) limited orbital haemorrhage after third-time revisional orbital decompression.

Further reading

Bartalena L, Marcocci C, Bogazzi F *et al.* Relation between therapy for hyperthyroidism and the course of Graves' ophthalmopathy. *New Engl J Med* 1998; **338**:73–8.

Burch HB, Wartofsky L. Graves' ophthalmopathy: current concepts regarding pathogenesis and management. *Endocrinology Rev* 1993; **14**:747–93.

Char DH. *Thyroid eye disease* (3rd ed.) Boston: Butterworth-Heinemann, 1997.

Claridge KG, Ghabrial R, Davis G *et al.* Combined radiotherapy and medical immunosuppression in the management of thyroid eye disease. *Eye* 1997; **11**:717–22.

Consensus of an ad hoc committee. Classification of eye changes of Graves' disease. *Thyroid* 1992; **2**:235–6.

Fatourechi V, Garrity JA, Bartley GB, Bergstralh EJ, DeSanto LW, Gorman CA. Graves' ophthalmopathy. Results of transantral orbital decompression performed primarily for cosmetic indications. *Ophthalmology* 1994; **101**:938–42.

Garrity JA, Fatourechi V, Bergstralh EJ *et al.* Results of transantral orbital decompression in 428 patients with severe Graves' ophthalmopathy. *Am J Ophthalmol* 1993; **116**:533–47.

Hales JB, Rundle FF. Ocular changes in Graves' disease: a long term follow-up study. QJM 1960; **29**:113–9.

Kalmann R, Mourits MP, van der Pol JP, Koornneef L. Coronal approach for rehabilitative orbital decompression in Graves' ophthalmopathy. *Br J Ophthalmol* 1997; **81**:41–5.

Lyons CJ, Rootman J. Orbital decompression for disfiguring exophthalmos in thyroid orbitopathy. *Ophthalmology* 1994; **101**:223–30.

McCord CD Jr. Orbital decompression for Graves' disease; exposure through lateral canthal and inferior fornix incision. *Ophthalmology* 1981; **88**:533–41.

Metson R, Dallow RL, Shore JW. Endoscopic orbital decompression. *Laryngoscope* 1994; **104**:950–7.

Mourits MP, Koornneef L, Wiersinga WM, Prummel MF, Berghout A, van der Gaag R. Clinical criteria for the assessment of disease activity in Graves' ophthalmopathy; a novel approach. *Br J Ophthalmol* 1989; **73**:639–44.

Mourits MP, Koornneef L, Wiersinga WM, Prummel MF, Berghout A, van der Gaag R. Orbital decompression for Graves' ophthalmopathy by inferomedial, by inferomedial plus lateral, and by coronal approach. *Ophthalmology* 1990; **97**:636–41.

Naniaris N, Hurwitz JJ, Chen JC, Wortzman G. Correlation between computed tomography and magnetic resonance imaging in Graves' orbitopathy. *Can J Ophthalmol* 1994; **29**:9–19.

Olivari, N. Transpalpebral decompression of endocrine ophthalmopathy (Graves' disease) by removal of intraorbital fat: experience with 147 operations over 5 years. *Plast Reconstr Surg* 1979; **87**:627–41.

Perros P, Crombie AL, Kendall-Taylor P. Natural history of thyroid associated ophthalmopathy. *Clin Endocrinol Oxf* 1995; **42**:45–54.

Prummel MF, Wiersinga WM. Medical management of Graves' ophthalmopathy. *Thyroid* 1995; **5**:231–4.

Prummel MF, Wiersinga WM, Mourits MP *et al.* Effect of abnormal thyroid function on severity of Graves' ophthalmopathy. *Arch Intern Med* 1990; **150**:1098–101.

Shine B, Fells P, Edwards OM, Weetman OP. Association between Graves' ophthalmopathy and smoking. *Lancet* 1990; **335**:1261–3.

Tagami T, Tanaka K, Sugawa H, *et al.* High-dose intravenous steroid pulse therapy in thyroid-associated opthalmopathy. *Endocr J* 1996; **43**:689–99.

Trokel S, Kazim M, Moore S. Orbital fat removal. Decompression for Graves' orbitopathy. *Ophthalmology* 1993; **100**:674–82.

Werner SC. Classification of changes in Graves' disease. *J Clin Endocrinol Metab* 1969; **29**:982–9.

Wulc A, Popp JC, Bartlett SP. Lateral wall advancement in orbital decompression. *Ophthalmology* 1990; **97**:1358–69.

12 Benign orbital disease

Christopher J McLean

Benign orbital diseases, for many of which the clinical history and examination findings are diagnostic, cover a wide spectrum. The incidence varies with age but, although obviously dependent upon referral patterns, in childhood the most common benign lesions are dermoid and epidermoid cysts (6–37%), capillary haemangiomas (8–13%) and trauma (7%), whereas adult series are typically dominated by thyroid orbitopathy (Chapter 11), orbital trauma (Chapter 14) and orbital infections.

Benign cystic anomalies of the orbit

Orbital cysts generally arise from epithelium sequestered within the orbit during embryological development, by implantation after trauma or due to expansion of epithelial-lined sinus lesions into the orbit.

Dermoid and epidermoid cysts

These lesions arise from surface epithelium implanted at sites of embryological folding and, if situated anteriorly within the orbit, are commonly noted soon after birth. Due to the accumulation of epithelial debris and sebaceous oil in the lumen of the cyst, the cysts slowly enlarge and leakage of the contents into the surrounding tissues may cause marked inflammation – with deeper dermoid cysts tending to present in this fashion. A dermoid cyst contains dermal structures (hairs, sebaceous glands), whereas more rarely there is only an epithelial (epidermoid cyst) or a conjunctival lining (conjunctival dermoid).

Implantation cysts may arise and develop in a similar fashion to congenital dermoids, but do not respect the characteristic anatomic sites of the latter and will generally present in patients with a past history of periocular trauma.

The commonest dermoid cysts are firm and smooth, mobile preseptal masses overlying the supero-temporal quadrant of the orbit and, less commonly, the supero-nasal quadrant. Many cysts have a variable periosteal attachment near the underlying fronto-zygomatic or fronto-ethmoidal sutures, but occasionally the dermoid will pass into or through defects in the neighbouring bone. In some cases the dermoid is incompletely separated from the skin surface and presents as a chronically inflamed and discharging sinus (Figure 12.1).

A clinically characteristic lesion presenting in childhood does not require radiological investigation if anteriorly situated and mobile. Likewise, fixed anterior masses do not necessitate imaging, provided the orbital surgeon is adequately experienced to follow the lesion to its limits – if necessary within the orbital depths. Deep orbital dermoids, often presenting as orbital inflammation or proptosis, require thin-slice CT with bone

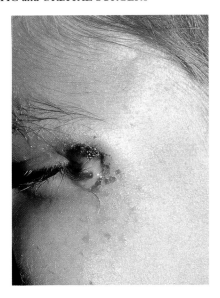

Figure 12.1 Dermoid cyst in communication with the skin, presenting as a discharging fistula.

windows to show associated clefts or canals in the bone (Figure 12.2); MRI is a poor investigation for these orbital abnormalities. CT will often show a smooth, "scalloped" erosion of the neighbouring bone as a result of pressure from the mass, although this is a non-specific sign suggesting a longstanding benign orbital lesion.

All cysts develop inflammatory changes and should be removed, generally at preschool age before childhood trauma encourages rupture.

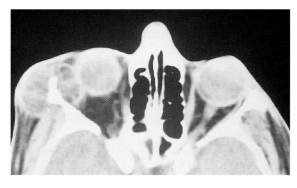

Figure 12.2 CT scan showing orbital and temporalis fossa components of a dermoid cyst, with associated bone changes.

They are excised through an incision hidden in the upper lid skin-crease or brow line and it is important to divide tissues right down to the cyst (there being a tendency to dissect a plane too far from the surface of the cyst) and then follow the plane by blunt dissection; in some cases it is necessary to remove some of the underlying periosteum or follow the lesion into or through the orbital walls.

Deep orbital dermoids often involve the greater wing of the sphenoid and may require lateral orbitotomy or complicated anterior orbitotomy for their removal.

Rupture of the cyst during surgery may lead to a marked post operative inflammation and any spilt contents should be removed. Incomplete excision of the epithelial lining will lead to recurrent inflammation with formation of a discharging cutaneous fistula to the operative site.

Dermolipoma

Although dermolipomas are not cystic, they are conveniently classified with dermoid cysts as they arise from cutaneous epithelium sequestered within the conjunctival recesses – typically laterally and occasionally associated with a minor clefting of the outer canthus or with Goldenhar's syndrome. The abnormal epithelium, which often bears hairs and sebaceous glands that cause chronic conjunctivitis, is associated with localised prenatal formation of cutaneous-type fat, which is evident as an underlying bright yellow mass. The differential diagnosis is subconjunctival fat prolapse, which tends to present in obese adults and is not associated with an abnormal conjunctival surface.

Dermolipomas require removal if they are causing chronic conjunctivitis or if easily visible at the palpebral aperture. Excision should be performed under the operating microscope as this aids preservation of all except the abnormal epithelium and reduces the risk of damage to the lacrimal gland ductules. To avoid adherence between the lateral rectus and the orbital rim, only fat anterior to the rim should be removed and this abnormal cutaneous fat has a subtle plane of dissection free from the normal orbital fat.

Incautious excision of dermolipomas is a source of medico-legal cases, as there is a significant risk of damage to the lacrimal gland ductules, restriction of eye movements and ptosis if the lesions are not managed properly.

Paranasal sinus mucocoeles

Mucocoeles, most commonly in the anterior ethmoid and frontal sinuses, are slowly-enlarging, mucus-filled, cystic lesions that arise from paranasal sinus mucosa and gradually encroach into the orbit; occasionally the contents of a mucocoele become infected, which may lead to orbital cellulitis. Most mucocoeles will present with a gradual displacement of the globe and proptosis (Figure 12.3), although those of the maxillary sinus may lead to collapse of the orbital floor and secondary enophthalmos.

The CT appearance of a mucocoele is a cystic cavity smoothly expanding the bone of a paranasal sinus and necessary with patchy thinning or loss of bone. T1- and T2-weighted MR images can show a wide variation in signal intensities due to continuing changes in the contents of the mucocoele.

Severe acute sinusitis or orbital cellulitis requires admission for intravenous antibiotic

therapy and drainage of the orbital abscess if threatening vision. Once the infection has been shown to be under control, the mucocoele and other sinus disease should receive definitive treatment under the care of an otorhinolaryngologist. In general, treatment involves removal of the mucocoele lining and re-establishment of a new drainage pathway for the affected sinus.

Orbital cellulitis secondary to infected mucocoeles may lead to an orbital abscess or the formation of a transcutaneous fistula, typically in the medial aspect of the upper eyelid. Late presentation of mucocoeles within the sphenoid or posterior ethmoid sinuses can lead to compressive optic neuropathy and irreversible visual loss.

Cranial and orbital anomalies

Microphthalmos with cyst

Microphthalmos with cyst arises from incomplete closure of the fissure in the optic vesicle, with formation of a cyst below a microphthalmic globe. The cysts can vary greatly in size and may slowly enlarge.

Small cysts can be left and may be in communication with the vitreous cavity. Large cysts are cosmetically unacceptable, cause excessive orbital bony expansion, and generally need to be removed together with the microphthalmic globe; a ball implant can be placed at the same operation and, in all cases, a suitable fornix conformer must be placed (Chapter 9).

Excision of small or moderately sized orbital cysts may retard orbital growth and lead to problems with prosthetics fitting later in life. Ball implantation can, on occasion, be difficult due to abnormal extraocular musculature.

Cephalocoeles

Congenital clefts of the skull, with herniation of intracranial contents, leads to

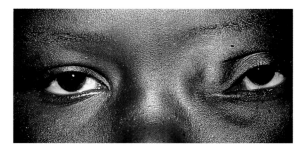

Figure 12.3   Outward displacement of the left globe due to ethmoidal mucocoele.

cephalocoeles: the herniating contents can be meninges (meningocoeles), brain tissues (encephalocoeles), or both tissues (meningo-encephalocoeles). When involving the orbit, they often present in childhood as fullness above the medial canthus, this swelling increasing with straining or bending. Some patients with orbital encephalocoeles will have neurofibromatosis and the association of colobomatous optic disc with basal encephalocoele is known as "morning glory syndrome".

Direct coronal CT scanning is best for identifying the skull base deformity that always accompanies orbital meningocoeles and encephalocoeles.

Orbital cephalocoeles are removed as part of the major reconstruction in affected children, who often have multiple cranio-facial anomalies, and defects within the sphenoid bone are hard to correct compared to those of the frontal bone.

Benign vascular anomalies of the orbit

Many vascular anomalies, such as varices, lymphangiomas and cavernous haemangiomas, are probably present from birth but may only become manifest in early adulthood.

Capillary haemangiomas

Capillary haemangiomas occur in 1–2% of infants and are more common in females and children of low birth weight; most appear soon after birth, can enlarge dramatically and then undergo a spontaneous involution – with 75% resolving within five years. Involvement is usually unilateral and the intradermal eyelid lesions are bright red and dimpled (so called, "strawberry naevus"; Figure 12.4), whereas the deeper orbital lesions have a blue colouration and spongy texture; both may increase slightly in size with crying or straining.

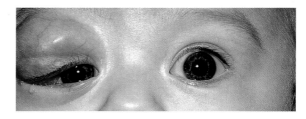

Figure 12.4 Orbital capillary haemangioma in an infant.

The rapid growth of a deep orbital capillary haemangioma may mimic the highly malignant rhabdomyosarcoma and it is important to be aware of this differential diagnosis; Doppler ultrasonography will, however, show high reflectivity and vessels with very high flow-rate (over 50cm/s) within the capillary haemangioma. CT scan is rarely necessary, but typically shows an irregular, poorly defined lesion with marked contrast enhancement.

Affected children should be monitored for impairment of visual development, being refracted when at an age suitable for spectacle correction of anisometropia or marked astigmatism. If the child is tending to develop an amblyopic eye, then appropriate corrective measures should be taken to maintain vision and consideration be given to treating the lesion.

Many capillary haemangiomas will regress rapidly, or their growth be slowed, by injecting them with corticosteroids under general anaesthesia; a useful regime being 40mg depomedrone in the lesion and 4mg soluble dexamethasone around the lesion, this being repeated at six-weekly intervals for two further sessions. Before injecting, the plunger must be drawn back and, if blood is present, the needle should be resited to avoid intravascular injection.

Systemic interferon has been used to treat steroid-resistant, life-threatening capillary haemangiomas, but the systemic side effects render it inapplicable to orbital lesions. Because of the risk of major haemorrhage, surgery is not recommended for most capillary haemangiomas.

When the haemangioma has regressed, it may be necessary to remove redundant atrophic eyelid skin or correct ptosis resulting from disinsertion of the levator muscle aponeurosis.

The complications of intralesional steroid injections are necrosis of the skin overlying the capillary haemangioma, and atrophy of subcutaneous fat or dermis. Rarely growth retardation and blindness have been reported with this therapy.

Cavernous haemangiomas

Cavernous haemangioma is the most common benign orbital tumour of adults and may be a developmental hamartoma that presents late in life, typically in the fourth or fifth decades, with gradually increasing painless proptosis. It is usually solitary and lies in the retrobulbar space, thereby causing axial proptosis, induced presbyopia, choroidal folds and optic disc congestion. There is often a global reduction in the extremes of eye movement.

CT scanning reveals a well defined, round intraconal lesion that commonly displaces the optic nerve medially and, due to a very slow blood flow, shows a very slow and patchy contrast enhancement (Figure 12.5). Some haemangiomas are wedged in the orbital apex

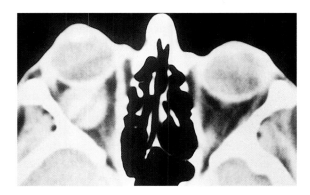

Figure 12.5 CT scan appearance of well-defined intraconal cavernous haemangioma; the differential diagnosis being the rarer orbital neurilemmoma.

and these tend to present early due to optic neuropathy. On MRI scanning, cavernous haemangiomas are hypointense to fat on T1-weighted images and isointense to vitreous and hyperintense to fat and vitreous on T2-weighted images.

Patients with asymptomatic tumours, discovered by chance on imaging for other reasons, can be monitored for orbital signs and many presumed haemangiomas show minimal change over many years. Indications for removal include optic neuropathy, proptosis and diplopia.

Lateral orbitotomy with intact excision of the tumour is usually required, as many haemangiomas are large and intraconal. The tumour typically is like a purple plum and contains large blood-filled cystic spaces.

Method for lateral orbitotomy

An upper eyelid skin-crease incision is extended laterally to about 1cm below the lateral canthus (Figure 12.6a) and the tissues opened to the supero-lateral orbital rim. The periosteum is incised 6mm outside the rim, from the lateral one-third of the upper rim to the level of the zygomatic arch, the origin of the temporalis muscle separated from the bone over its antero-superior 2cm, and the periosteal incision extended backwards over the zygomatic arch (Figure 12.6b). The periosteum is elevated over the rim of the orbit and separated from the inner aspect of the lateral wall, with particular care being taken to cauterise and divide any bridging vessels. Two parallel saw cuts are made, in the coronal plane, at the upper and lower ends of the lateral osteotomy, drill holes placed either side of the cuts and the inner aspect of the lateral wall fragment weakened 1cm behind the rim, using a burr; the fragment is then broken away and trimmed, to be swung outwards on the temporalis muscle (Figure 12.6c), and the periosteum opened to provide access for the intraorbital procedure.

After achieving intraorbital haemostasis, a vacuum drain is placed within the intraconal

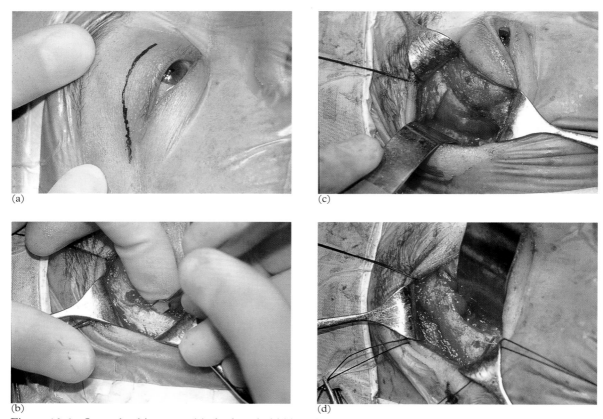

Figure 12.6 Lateral orbitotomy: (a) the largely hidden skin incision; (b) the periosteum being raised over the lateral rim; (c) the lateral wall hinged outwards on temporalis muscle; (d) the bone fixed in position with a 4/0 absorbable suture.

space and passed out through the skin overlying the temporalis fossa. The bone is swung medially into the correct position and fixed into place with a 4/0 absorbable suture passed through the drill holes (Figure 12.6d). The deep subcutaneous tissues over the outer canthus and further laterally are closed with a 4/0 or 5/0 absorbable suture and the skin incision closed with a running 6/0 nylon suture.

The patient should be nursed upright after surgery and it is important that any severe or increasing pain is reported. Where pain is severe or increasing, the vision in the affected eye and the state of the orbit should be checked; a very tense orbit with markedly decreased vision, a relative afferent pupillary defect and loss of eye movements, suggests

accumulation of orbital haemorrhage and this may lead to irreversible visual loss. If this emergency appears to be developing, the drain should be moved slightly to see if drainage of fluid from the orbit occurs; if this does not succeed, the operative site should be reopened at the "bedside", without delay, and any accumulation of blood allowed to drain.

The vacuum drain is removed when active fluid drainage has ceased (usually 12–18 hours after surgery) and post operative systemic anti-inflammatory medications at high dosage are useful, particularly where there has been manipulation in the region of the superior orbital fissure or optic nerve. The patient should refrain from vigorous exercise for 10 days after surgery, normal ocular ductions encouraged and the skin suture removed at one week.

Complications

Excision of cavernous haemangiomas is curative, although the induced hyperopia and choroidal folds do not resolve in all cases.

Complications with removal of cavernous haemangiomas are more related to the lateral orbitotomy and the need to displace tissues to reach the tumour. It is common to get a transient weakness of ocular ductions, particularly abduction, and this typically improves over several weeks. Motor neuropraxias, which may recover over many months, are also fairly common with surgery near the orbital apex and superior orbital fissure; post operative mydriasis, probably due to denervation at the ciliary ganglion, is relatively common and may be permanent. Blindness due to optic nerve compression or ischaemia is a distinct risk with any surgery involving the posterior half of the orbit.

Orbital varices and lymphangiomas

Orbital varices and lymphangiomas are a spectrum of congenital low-pressure vascular malformations with venous-type channels that typically are unilateral and may involve ipsilateral parts of the face and brain, as well as the orbit.

In the absence of lymphatics from the human orbit, the term "lymphangioma" appears to be a misnomer. It serves, however, to emphasise an important clinical distinction between the two groups of low-pressure vascular anomalies that occur in various admixtures within different patients. Varices are largely blood-filled and generally in free communication with the normal low-pressure vascular system of the orbit, whereas "lymphangiomas" are largely isolated from the venous system and have a much greater component of inflammatory infiltration.

Whilst an ophthalmologist should supervise the day-to-day management of visual development of children with these malformations, the surgical management is an ophthalmic specialist field, being both difficult and liable to complication.

Lymphangiomas

These typically present between the ages of 6 and 10 years, as haemorrhage within cystic spaces deep in the orbit (so-called "chocolate cysts") or as superficial lesions with multi-loculated cysts of the conjunctiva or lid margin; proptosis and displacement of the globe occur as deep components enlarge. An increase in the size of lymphangiomas during respiratory infections, possibly due to lymphoid hypertrophy or vascular congestion, is frequently noted with these malformations. Orbital CT scan will demonstrate irregular, multi-loculated cystic opacities within the normal (but displaced) structures of an expanded orbit. Ultrasonography often shows acoustically empty cystic spaces.

An attempt should be made to optimise visual development in the eye affected by the orbital malformation, with treatment of anisometropia or astigmatism, and occlusion of the unaffected eye where necessary. Complete surgical excision of orbital lymphangiomas is, effectively, impossible and would be liable to damage the interspersed normal orbital structures. Surgery is, therefore, reserved for debulking the lesion anterior to the equator of the globe to improve cosmesis – for example, where there is prolapse of abnormal tissues through the palpebral aperture. Otherwise deep components may be drained or resected where there is gross displacement of the globe or compressive optic neuropathy.

Despite all efforts to maintain visual development, large lymphangiomas almost inevitably result in some degree of amblyopia. Compressive optic neuropathy may result from large intraorbital haemorrhages and there is a risk to all orbital structures during surgery to drain or excise these lesions.

Orbital varices

Although very rarely secondary to orbital arterio-venous communication, almost all varices are primary, congenital, low-pressure malformations that typically present in the second or third decade. Many patients will first notice intermittent proptosis, occasionally painful, on bending or straining and this may be simulated, during examination, by the Valsalva manoeuvre; in some cases the varices are non-distensible and may present with a sudden onset of painful proptosis due to haemorrhage within the varix.

Orbital enlargement on CT scan is common with varices and the serpiginous opacities of the malformation (Figure 12.7) may show phleboliths, small flecks of calcification within intravascular thrombi. Management of orbital varices is similar to that for the allied lymphangiomas, with maintenance of visual development and limited surgical intervention for anterior lesions, or large malformations causing visual problems or a major interruption of life-style; surgical resection carries, however, a significant risk of major haemorrhage and blindness.

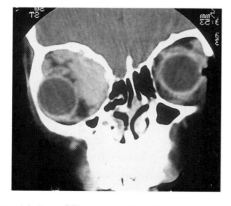

Figure 12.7   CT scan of orbital varices in an enlarged orbit.

Orbital arterio-venous communications

High-pressure arterio-venous communications within the orbit are characterised by pulsatile proptosis and chemosis, a global reduction in eye movements and dilation of episcleral veins with raised intraocular pressure. The high pressure and flow within the orbital veins may result from an arterio-venous shunt within the orbit or in the anterior part of the intracranial circulation.

Intraorbital arterio-venous malformations

Branches of both the internal and external carotid arteries commonly supply orbital arterio-venous malformations, either spontaneous or post-traumatic. CT scan typically shows unilateral proptosis with mild enlargement of all extraocular muscles, a diffuse increase in opacity of the orbital fat and widespread engorgement of tortuous orbital vessels. Orbital Doppler ultrasonography will show widespread engorgement of vessels and arterial waveforms within veins – particularly the superior ophthalmic vein where there may be reversal of the (normally posteriorly-directed) flow.

Super-selective angiography of branches of the internal and external carotid arteries is required, with embolisation of the vessels supplying the abnormal communication. Resection of remaining abnormal vessels may be undertaken, although surgery for these lesions tends to be difficult and the results somewhat unsatisfactory.

Dural shunts

Dural shunts commonly present with a chronic "red eye" (Figure 12.8) and are due to a spontaneous fistula between a minor dural vessel and the cavernous venous sinus. CT scan shows orbital changes similar to those of an intraorbital arterio-venous communication

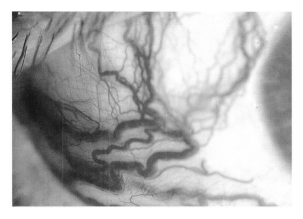

Figure 12.8   Dilated episcleral veins due to a low-flow dural arterio-venous shunt.

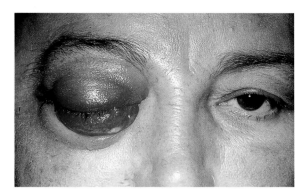

Figure 12.9   Gross chemosis, proptosis and vascular dilation due to high-flow post-traumatic carotico-cavernous fistula.

but, in addition, there may be engorgement of the ipsilateral cavernous sinus and possibly also some subtle changes in the contralateral cavernous sinus and orbit. Doppler ultrasonography is, again, valuable in the diagnosis of these lesions.

Most low-flow dural arterio-venous shunts will resolve spontaneously over many months and treatment (with arteriography and possible embolisation) is required only where a high-flow fistula is causing visual failure, unacceptable proptosis, or persistent severe proptosis.

Carotico-cavernous fistula

These high-pressure, high-flow communications generally present with acute proptosis, eyelid swelling, chemosis with engorged episcleral vessels, raised intraocular pressure, retinal haemorrhages and ocular ischaemia; in some cases palsies of the third and sixth cranial nerves may be present. They arise spontaneously in atheromatous individuals, with rupture of the intracavernous internal carotid artery into the venous sinus, or occur after severe head injury (Figure 12.9).

Radiological imaging shows a more extreme version of the changes seen with low-flow dural shunts and arteriography is required in most cases. Balloon occlusion of the fistula is effective in 90% of cases and has a low morbidity.

Benign lacrimal gland disease

The lacrimal gland is liable to inflammation, cysts and benign tumours, but these conditions can present in a similar fashion to malignancy and this complicates the clinical management of these patients. Inappropriate management of benign conditions can lead to serious consequences – as with, for example, malignant recurrence after biopsy of a benign pleomorphic adenoma.

Dacryocoele (Dacryops)

Dacryocoele is a retention cyst of a gland ductule and often presents in young adults, with a variable swelling in the supero-temporal conjunctival fornix and bursts of apparent lacrimation. The clinical diagnosis is absolute and imaging is not required.

Microsurgical opening of the cyst, to allow free drainage of the affected ductule, is indicated only where the cyst is large and persistent. Surgery should be with an operating microscope and the greatest of care taken to avoid damage to the normal lacrimal gland ductules – for fear of a post operative dry eye.

131

Very rarely the affected ductule will become infected with Actinomyces, this causing a slightly inflamed and chronically discharging eye.

Pleomorphic adenoma

Pleomorphic adenomas account for about 5% of all orbital tumours, 25% of lacrimal fossa masses and 50% of all epithelial tumours of the lacrimal gland. Most affect the orbital lobe and become evident in the fourth and fifth decade as a slow onset of painless proptosis and infero-medial displacement of the globe; the much rarer palpebral lobe lesions present in young people with a shorter history of a hard, mobile mass above the lateral part of the upper tarsus.

Orbital lobe tumours show a smooth expansion of the lacrimal gland fossa by an oval lesion in which calcification is rare, the mass causing displacement of orbital structures and often flattening of the globe (Figure 12.10); it is unusual for these tumours, even when large, to extend anterior to the orbital rim. In contrast, the rare palpebral lobe tumours show a normal gland with an enlarged, rounded anterior surface extending outside the orbital rim on CT scan.

The key to treatment of pleomorphic adenomas is recognition, on the basis of

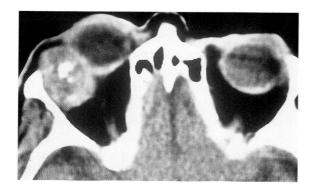

Figure 12.10 CT scan of a typical pleomorphic adenoma, showing displacement and flattening of the globe by a round lesion that may cause scalloping of the bone in the lacrimal fossa.

clinical history and radiological signs, with avoidance of biopsy. Because of the long-term risk of spontaneous malignant transformation, tumours of the orbital lobe should be excised intact through a lateral orbitotomy and breach of the "pseudocapsule" of compressed tissues avoided; to this end, the tumour is handled at all times with a malleable retractor and not with any form of forceps.

Palpebral lobe pleomorphic adenomas, sometimes mistaken for large chalazia and curetted, are excised intact through an upper eyelid skin-crease incision.

Breach of the pseudocapsule of these tumours risks a pervasive recurrence of tumour (sometimes malignant) throughout the orbit, this necessitating orbital exenteration. Although there are advocates of fine-needle aspiration biopsy of these tumours, there is no logical reason for undertaking this in the presence of clinically and radiologically characteristic disease.

Keratitis sicca can be troublesome in a few cases, although the incidence of this condition is lower with preservation of the palpebral lobe during excision of these tumours. It is treated with topical lubricants and, where necessary, occlusion of the lacrimal drainage canaliculi.

Dacryoadenitis

The lacrimal gland may be affected by an acute polymorphic inflammation, which may be due to bacterial infection, or a chronic, predominantly lymphocytic, dacryoadenitis which may be due to underlying systemic diseases such as sarcoid or Wegener's granulomatosis.

Acute dacryoadenitis presents with painful, red swelling of the upper eyelid – with an "S"-shaped ptosis (Figure 12.11) – and tenderness of the underlying lacrimal gland; systemic malaise is unusual.

Painless swelling of one or both lacrimal glands is the usual manifestation of chronic dacryoadenitis and the gland often shows

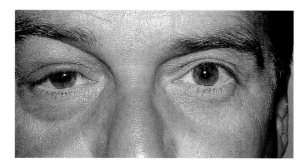

Figure 12.11   Slightly "S"-shaped lateral ptosis due to lacrimal gland enlargement.

diffuse enlargement on CT, with extension of changes outside the limits of the gland and with moulding of the abnormal tissue around the globe (Figure 12.12) – unlike the compressive flattening of the globe seen with pleomorphic adenoma.

Although most acute dacryoadenitis is probably not bacterial, it is usual to treat such cases with a course of systemic antibiotics and non-steroidal anti-inflammatory medications. If inflammation persists or worsens, orbital

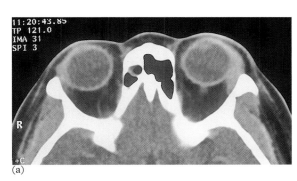

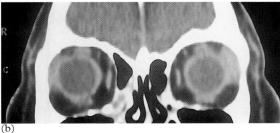

Figure 12.12   Diffuse enlargement of the lacrimal gland on CT scan, due to dacryoadenitis: (a) axial view, (b) coronal view.

CT scan should be performed with a view to surgical drainage of an abscess or biopsy of a lacrimal gland mass. The patient should be followed for several months, until there is clear evidence of resolution of any mass; if there is a persistent lacrimal gland mass, the patient should be scanned with a view to biopsy, as malignancy of the lacrimal gland may present as subacute dacryoadenitis.

Chronic dacryoadenitis requires CT scan of the orbit, chest x ray and blood tests for sarcoid and other systemic inflammatory diseases. If CT demonstrates lacrimal gland enlargement with moulding to the globe, then biopsy is indicated. If the mass is fixed at the orbital rim and palpable, then biopsy may be achieved under local anaesthesia, but otherwise general anaesthesia should be used as it can be difficult to locate mobile intraorbital masses under local anaesthesia.

General method for anterior orbitotomy and incisional biopsy

A skin incision is placed in a suitably hidden position, generally the upper eyelid skin-crease or the lower eyelid "tear trough", and for most incisional biopsies should be about 3cm long. The underlying orbicularis muscle is cauterised and divided at the midpoint of the skin incision, the points of a pair of scissors inserted through the defect and the scissors opened widely along the line of the muscle fibres, to separate them by blunt dissection; any remaining bridging tissues are diathermied and divided to reveal the underlying orbital septum. The septum is likewise divided along the line of incision, to expose the orbital fat, and the direction of the mass to be biopsied ascertained by analysis of the imaging and by palpation.

A closed pair of blunt-tipped scissors is gently directed through the orbital fat towards the site to be biopsied and the scissors opened widely to reveal the depths of the tissues; before withdrawing the scissors, a 12–16mm malleable retractor is inserted alongside the opened scissors to maintain the plane and depth of exploration. This manoeuvre is then repeated until the abnormal tissue is reached, the surgical assistant maintaining as large a space as possible with the use of a pair of malleable retractors. Meticulous haemostasis is essential, as it can otherwise be almost impossible to recognise subtly abnormal orbital tissues – such as oedematous or infiltrated orbital fat.

When the abnormal tissue is located, which can be very difficult, then a relatively large biopsy should be taken using a number 11 blade; the tissue should preferably be gripped once only, to avoid crush artefact, with a single larger piece being more diagnostic than small fragments.

Bipolar cautery should be used to establish complete haemostasis and the orbicularis and skin closed with a running 6/0 nylon suture; if the biopsy site is post-equatorial, then a drain (corrugated or vacuum) should be placed. The drain is generally removed on the day after biopsy and the skin/muscle suture removed at seven to ten days.

Severe acute dacryoadenitis may be accompanied by a marked secondary keratitis and, if bacterial, may rarely form an abscess alongside the gland. Chronic dacryoadenitis typically results in loss of glandular tissue and secondary fibrosis, with a sicca syndrome in occasional cases.

Benign orbital inflammatory disease

Dacryoadenitis forms just one class of orbital inflammation, but any orbital tissue may become inflamed either due to a specific aetiology or without a known cause. Scleritis and episcleritis are other subgroups of orbital inflammation that are discussed elsewhere.

Thyroid orbitopathy is a very specific form of orbital inflammation and is presented in Chapter 11.

Infective orbital cellulitis

Bacterial orbital infections are common and the age of the patient and site of origin help to indicate the likely organism and guide the selection of antibiotic therapy.

Preseptal infections generally arise from infected chalazia or insect bites and the eye remains uninflamed, with no chemosis, no proptosis and normal movements. Treatment is with an appropriate systemic antibiotic for soft-tissue cellulitis – such as a broad-spectrum cephalosporin – and review; drainage of a meibomian abscess will aid rapid resolution.

True orbital cellulitis (post-septal infection) presents with fever, systemic illness, periorbital swelling with proptosis, a red eye with chemosis and restricted eye movements (Figure 12.13). Optic neuropathy is present in more severe cases, being a sign of rising intraorbital pressure, and the onset of meningism or central neurological signs may herald the very serious complication of cavernous sinus thrombosis. In many cases there will be a history of antecedent upper respiratory tract infection or, in adults, a history of chronic sinus disease or dental infection. The most commonly identified bacteria are *Staphylococcus aureus*, *Streptococcus* species and, in children, also *Haemophilus influenzae*.

True infective orbital cellulitis is an emergency and requires immediate intravenous

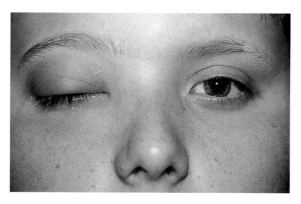

Figure 12.13 Orbital cellulitis in a child with persistent fever after coryza.

antibiotics; these should be given on clinical suspicion alone and their administration should not, under any circumstances, be delayed whilst arranging imaging or other investigations. Appropriate antibiotics should be at suitable dosage and active against the common organisms: a typical adult might receive Cefuroxime 1·5g every 8 hours (the child receiving a reduced dosage), along with Metronidazole 500mg every 8 hours in patients over the age of about 15.

When intravenous antibiotics have been given, thin slice CT of the orbits and sinuses will be required to demonstrate the likely source of infection and whether there is a localised collection of pus in the orbit or subperiosteal spaces. Once the orbital infection is controlled, with stabilisation or improvement in orbital status, then the patient should be referred for urgent treatment of the underlying sinus disease by an otorhinolaryngologist.

Where there is failing vision due to rising orbital pressure, the loss of vision can progress rapidly and lead to permanent blindness; in these cases, urgent drainage of the orbit is required and should be undertaken as an emergency. The site for primary exploration is indicated by the direction of globe displacement and drainage of pus and oedema (using, if urgency dictates, just local skin-infiltration anaesthesia) should be undertaken in the same fashion as drainage of an acute, sight-threatening haematoma (Chapter 14). When the focus of infection has been identified and drained, a corrugated drain should be left in place until there has been a clear improvement in orbital function.

If infective orbital cellulitis persists (or worsens after initial improvement) then the possibility of abscess formation, the presence of foreign material, reinfection with other bacteria, unusual organisms (fungi or tuberculosis) or a non-infective inflammatory cause (such as tumour necrosis) should be considered.

Severe complications of visual loss, cavernous sinus thrombosis and intracranial spread of infection may be secondary to late presentation, or progression due to inappropriate antibiotic selection at inadequate dosage; the latter situation should be preventable in most cases by close clinical monitoring.

Late abscess formation may require drainage to hasten resolution.

Orbital myositis

Typically presenting with a relatively sudden onset of orbital ache (worse on eye movement), ocular redness and diplopia, this condition is commonest in young women. The characteristic history and clinical signs – with pain worse when looking away from the field of action of the affected eye muscle – is sufficient to justify treatment with a non-steroidal anti-inflammatory drug, this typically relieving pain within a day. CT scan will demonstrate diffuse enlargement of one, or rarely more, eye muscles and, if severe, some "spillover" inflammatory changes in the surrounding orbital tissues.

Biopsy should be undertaken if the condition does not settle, with a view to treatment with systemic steroids or low-dose, lens-sparing irradiation of the retrobulbar tissues.

Patients may get recurrent episodes of myositis in various muscles and, in some cases, severe fibrosis of the affected muscles can result in a gross ocular deviation (Figure 12.14).

Idiopathic orbital inflammation

Idiopathic orbital inflammation occurs most commonly in the fourth and fifth decades, with no sex predilection, and is characterised by a polymorphous lymphoid infiltrate with a variable degree of fibrosis. It may present as an acute form with marked inflammation, or as a chronic form with a tendency to pain and fibrosis.

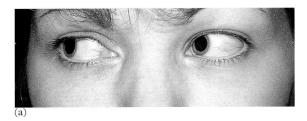

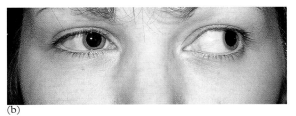

Figure 12.14   Restricted adduction and narrowing of the right palpebral aperture during adduction, due to fibrosis of the right lateral rectus after chronic myositis: (a) right gaze, (b) left gaze.

If inflammation is centred near the superior orbital fissure, a severe retrobulbar ache occurs with optic neuropathy, profound ophthalmoplegia and periorbital sensory loss, with almost no proptosis and relatively few inflammatory signs (Figure 12.15). This disease has a characteristically rapid and good response to high-dose systemic steroids, with resolution of pain and orbital signs within 24–48 hours.

CT scanning will demonstrate the extent of orbital involvement by the inflammation, with ill-defined opacity through the orbital fat and loss of definition of orbital structures. It is not, however, diagnostic and therefore biopsy is mandatory in all cases, except those with a characteristic history and response to treatment – namely orbital myositis and superior orbital fissure syndrome. The differential diagnoses for idiopathic orbital inflammation is extensive and includes infective orbital cellulitis, granulomatous orbital diseases (such as sarcoidosis or Wegener's granuloma), metastatic tumours and haematological malignancies, and appropriate systemic investigations (and biopsy) should be performed before starting systemic therapy.

Open biopsy at anterior orbitotomy will give the highest diagnostic yield and the

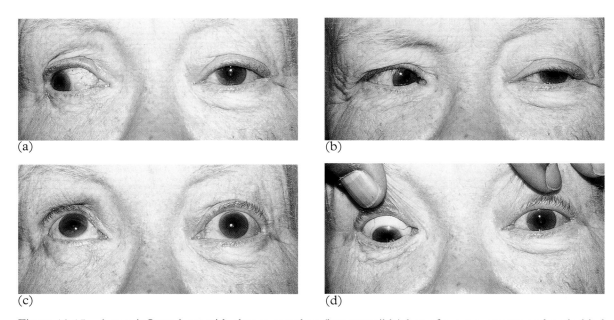

Figure 12.15   A non-inflamed eye with almost complete (but reversible) loss of eye movements and periorbital sensory impairment, due to orbital inflammation at the superior orbital fissure: (a) right gaze, (b) left gaze, (c) upgaze, (d) downgaze.

formed specimens are much more readily interpreted than those taken by aspiration needle biopsy; needle biopsy should, therefore, probably be used only for sampling lesions in patients with known carcinomatosis, in whom confirmation of a likely orbital metastasis is required prior to radiotherapy.

Treatment after biopsy is aimed at suppressing the inflammatory response with systemic corticosteroids or radiotherapy. In most instances, there is a good response to prednisolone 60–100mg per day (or 1mg/kg/day) and the dosage should be reduced towards 20mg daily within 3–4 weeks and more slowly thereafter. Radiotherapy to the retrobulbar tissues (generally 2000–2400cGy, in fractionated doses of 200cGy) may be valuable where there is a poor response to steroids, or where it is not possible to reduce the dosage to an acceptable level. Cytotoxic agents, such as cyclophosphamide, cyclosporin or methotrexate, have been used in recurrent and steroid-resistant orbital inflammation.

Benign neural and osseous lesions

Neurilemmomas (Schwannomas) typically present like cavernous haemangioma and have a similar scan appearance, and neurofibromas usually form a mass in the supraorbital nerve, with slowly progressive proptosis and hypoglobus; resection of these tumours, when causing loss of orbital function, is curative. In contrast, plexiform neurofibromas diffusely affect the anterior orbital tissues, especially in the upper eyelid and lacrimal gland, and resection is difficult and does not eliminate the disease.

Primary optic nerve tumours, either meningioma or glioma, are usually benign and present in childhood or young adults. Gliomas cause proptosis and mild visual loss and CT scan shows a fusiform enlargement of the optic nerve (Figure 12.16); MRI is particularly useful for demonstrating changes in the intracanalicular and intracranial portions of the nerve. Gliomas require neurosurgical resection, if progressing to threaten the optic chiasm, or orbital resection if causing gross proptosis. Optic nerve meningiomas do not cause significant proptosis, but profound visual failure due to impairment of optic nerve perfusion. CT scan typically shows a diffuse expansion of the optic nerve and, in some cases, calcification within the optic nerve sheath (Figure 12.17) and MRI may demonstrate a normal or small nerve passing through an enlarged sheath. Neurosurgical resection of optic nerve meningiomas may be considered in younger people, in whom the tumour appears to have a more active course and risks intracranial involvement.

There are many rare diseases that affect the orbital bones, but the commonest is sphenoid wing meningioma. This tends to present in middle age with chronic variable lid swelling, chemosis and mild proptosis. The CT scan shows hyperostosis of the greater wing of the sphenoid with en-plaque soft tissue on the lateral wall of the orbit, the temporalis fossa or the middle cranial fossa (Figure 12.18). Although a metastasis may very rarely present with a similar radiological appearance, the

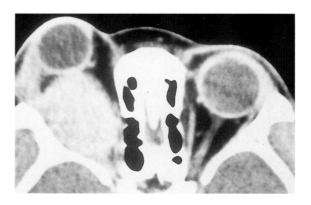

Figure 12.16 Optic nerve glioma causing fusiform enlargement of the nerve.

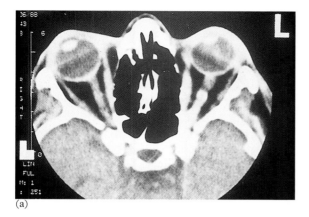

(a)

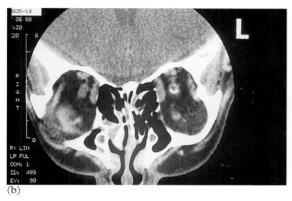

(b)

Figure 12.17 Elongated enlargement of the optic nerve, with linear calcification, due to primary optic nerve meningioma: (a) axial view, (b) coronal view.

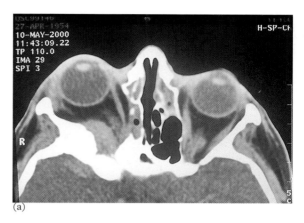

(a)

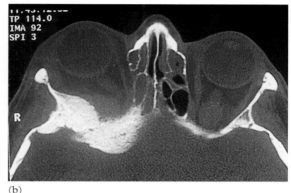

(b)

Figure 12.18 Hyperostosis and soft tissue mass of sphenoidal wing meningioma: (a) axial soft tissue, (b) bone CT scan windows.

clinical behaviour is different – with sphenoid wing meningioma progressing very slowly and usually not requiring any active treatment; biopsy is indicated if a rapid progression is suggestive of metastatic disease.

Further reading

Ferguson MP, McNab AA. Current treatment and outcome in orbital cellulitis. *Aust NZ J Ophthalmol* 1999; **27**:375–9.

Harris GJ. Subperiosteal abscess of the orbit: computed tomography and the clinical course. *Ophthal Plast Reconstr Surg* 1996; **12**:1–8.

Harris GJ, Logani SC. Eyelid crease incision for lateral orbitotomy. *Ophthal Plast Reconstr Surg* 1999; **15**:9–16.

Harris GJ, Sokol PJ, Bonavolonta G, De Conciliis C. An analysis of thirty cases of orbital lymphangiomas. Pathophysiologic considerations and management recommendations. *Ophthalmology* 1990; **97**:1583–92.

Katz BJ, Nerad JA. Ophthalmic manifestations of fibrous dysplasia: a disease of children and adults. *Ophthalmology* 1998; **105**:2207–15.

Lacey B, Chang W, Rootman J. Nonthyroid causes of extraocular muscle disease. *Surv Ophthalmol* 1999; **44**:187–213.

Lacey B, Rootman J, Marotta TR. Distensible venous malformations of the orbit: clinical and hemodynamic features and a new technique for management. *Ophthalmology* 1999; **106**:1197–209.

McNab AA, Wright JE. Cavernous haemangiomas of the orbit. *Aust NZ J Ophthalmol* 1989; **17**:337–45.

McNab AA, Wright JE. Lateral orbitotomy – a review. *Aust NZ J Ophthalmol* 1990; **18**:281–6.

McNab AA, Wright JE. Orbitofrontal cholesterol granuloma. *Ophthalmology* 1990; **97**:28–32.

McNab AA, Wright JE, Casswell AG. Clinical features and surgical management of dermolipomas. *Aust NZ J Ophthalmol* 1990; **18**:159–62.

Miszkiel KA, Sohaib SAA, Rose GE, Cree IA, Moseley IF. Radiological and clinicopathological features of orbital xanthogranuloma. *Br J Ophthalmol* 2000; **84**:251–8.

Nugent RA, Lapointe JS, Rootman J, Robertson WD, Graeb DA. Orbital dermoids: features on CT. *Radiology* 1987; **165**:475–8.

Rootman J. Why "orbital pseudotumour" is no longer a useful concept. *Br J Ophthalmol* 1998; **82**:339–40.

Rootman J, Hay E, Graeb D. Orbital adnexal lymphangiomas: a spectrum of hemodynamically isolated vascular hamartomas. *Ophthalmology* 1986; **93**:1558–70.

Rootman J, Kao SC, Graeb DA. Multidisciplinary approaches to complicated vascular lesions of the orbit. *Ophthalmology* 1992; **99**:1440–6.

Rootman J, McCarthy M, White V, Harris G, Kennerdell J. Idiopathic sclerosing inflammation of the orbit. A distinct clinicopathologic entity. *Ophthalmology* 1994; **101**:570–84.

Rose GE. Suspicion, speed, sufficiency and surgery: keys to the management of orbital infection. *Orbit* 1998; **17**:223–6.

Rose GE, Hoh B, Harrad RA, Hungerford JL. Intraocular malignant melanomas presenting with orbital inflammation. *Eye* 1993; **7**:539–41.

Rose GE, Wright JE. Isolated peripheral nerve sheath tumours of the orbit. *Eye* 1991; **5**:668–73.

Rose GE, Wright JE. Pleomorphic adenomas of the lacrimal gland. *Br J Ophthalmol* 1992; **76**:395–400.

Sathananthan N, Moseley IF, Rose GE, Wright JE. The frequency and significance of bone involvement in outer canthus dermoid cysts. *Br J Ophthalmol* 1993; **77**:789–94.

Shields JA, Kaden IH, Eagle RC Jr, Shields CL. Orbital dermoid cysts: clinicopathologic correlations, classification, and management. The 1997 Josephine E. Scheler Lecture. *Ophthal Plast Reconstr Surg* 1997; **13**:265–76.

Shields JA, Bakewell B, Augsberger JJ *et al*. Classification and incidence of space occupying lesions of the orbit: A survey of 645 biopsies. *Arch Ophthalmol* 1984; **102**:1606–11.

Sullivan TJ, Wright JE, Wulc AE, Garner A, Moseley IF, Sathananthan N. Haemangiopericytoma of the orbit. *Aust NZ J Ophthalmol* 1992; **20**:325–32.

Wright JE, McNab AA, McDonald WI. Primary optic nerve sheath meningioma. *Br J Ophthalmol* 1989; **73**:960–6.

Wright JE, McNab AA, McDonald WI. Optic nerve glioma and the management of optic nerve tumours of the young. *Br J Ophthalmol* 1989; **73**:967–74.

Wright JE, Sullivan TJ, Garner A, Wulc AE, Moseley IF. Orbital venous anomalies. *Ophthalmology* 1997; **104**:905–13.

13 Malignant orbital disease

Michael J Wearne

Malignant orbital disease, either primary or secondary, is rare but can affect all ages from infancy to old age. The possibility of malignant disease should, therefore, be entertained wherever there is a rapidly or relentlessly progressive disease, an inflammatory picture or where assumed non-malignant orbital disease does not display characteristic behaviour.

Malignant orbital disease in children

Although very rare, the very aggressive malignancies of rhabdomyosarcoma or neuroblastoma tend to present under the age of 10 years, the acute haematological malignancies within the first two decades and primary lacrimal gland malignancy has a peak incidence in the fourth decade.

Rhabdomyosarcoma

Rhabdomyosarcoma, with a peak incidence at age 7, is the commonest primary orbital malignancy of childhood and arises from pleuripotent mesenchyme that normally differentiates into striated muscle cells. Although rhabdomyosarcoma classically presents with signs of acute orbital cellulitis (Figure 13.1a), in some cases it is more insidious and mimics a benign process; a high index of suspicion is required for any unilateral orbital disease in childhood. At this age the main differential diagnosis for a

rapidly growing tumour mass is a deep orbital capillary haemangioma, although children with haemangiomas will often have other cutaneous vascular lesions.

The tumour mass may be located anywhere in the orbital soft tissues, most commonly in the supero-medial quadrant, and typically does *not* arise in the extraocular muscles. Orbital imaging will usually demonstrate a fairly well defined, round mass arising within the orbital fat and flattening the globe (Figure 13.1b),

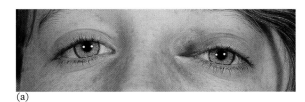
(a)

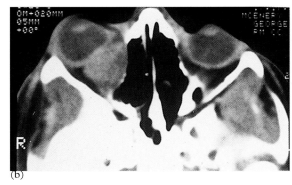
(b)

Figure 13.1 Childhood rhabdomyosarcoma may present as a rapidly growing orbital mass (a) or with inflammatory signs; (b) the rapidly progressive tumour may compress the globe and typically is not associated with muscle.

the tumour showing moderate contrast enhancement. Expansion of the adjacent thin childhood orbital bones is fairly common, but calcification of the tumour is rare.

Doppler ultrasonography may be helpful in differentiating capillary haemangiomas from rhabdomyosarcomas, the haemangiomas showing marked vascularity with very high flow-rates.

Urgent incisional biopsy, using an anterior transcutaneous or transconjunctival approach (Chapter 12), is required to confirm the diagnosis, although macroscopic excision may be possible for well-defined small tumours. On confirmation of diagnosis, a systemic evaluation, including whole-body CT scan and bone marrow biopsy, is required to look for metastatic disease.

The commonest variant of the tumour is the embryonal type, the alveolar is clinically aggressive with a bad prognosis, and the pleomorphic variant (the rarest) has the best prognosis. The 5-year survival is greater than 90% with local radiotherapy and adjuvant chemotherapy as the mainstay of treatment, although local resection of residual tumour (or orbital exenteration) may be needed in a few cases.

Long-term side-effects of orbital radiotherapy include cataract, dry eye with secondary corneal scarring, loss of skin appendages (lashes and brow hair), atrophy of orbital fat and, if performed in infancy, retardation of orbital bone growth. There is also a risk of late radiation-induced orbital malignancy, such as fibrosarcoma and osteosarcoma, and there may be an increased propensity to certain other primary tumours in adulthood.

Other malignancies

Neuroblastoma may present as rapidly progressive metastasis within the orbital soft tissues or bone (Figure 13.2), the clinical presentation being very similar to

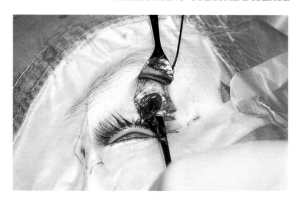

Figure 13.2 Neuroblastoma metastatic to the orbital rim in an infant.

rhabdomyosarcoma. Another childhood malignancy that may present with orbital inflammatory signs is acute myeloid leukaemia (Figure 13.3a); this is also known as "chloroma", the tumour tissue turning green on exposure to air (Figure 13.3b). Langerhans cell histiocytosis (of which there

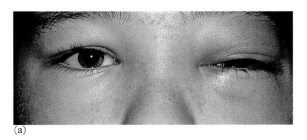

(a)

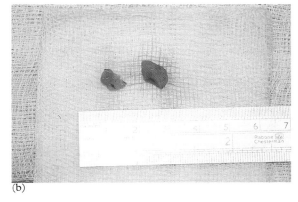

(b)

Figure 13.3 (a) Acute myeloid leukaemia presenting with persistent orbital cellulitis; (b) the tumour may be termed chloroma because the tissue turns green in air.

are three main variants) is a proliferative disease of Langerhans cells that may be malignant, although the variant found most commonly in children – eosinophilic granuloma – verges on a benign proliferation and is readily treated.

All of these childhood tumours require urgent biopsy, systemic investigation and chemotherapy with, in some cases, radiotherapy. Although prognosis for vision with most of the haematological malignancies is generally good there is a significant mortality, depending on pre-chemotherapy disease staging.

Malignant orbital diseases in adults

As with all cancers, orbital malignancy is more common in middle age and in the elderly and may be either primary disease arising in the orbit, secondary to spread from the sinuses, or metastatic from remote sites.

Lacrimal gland carcinoma

Adenoid cystic carcinoma, with a peak incidence in the fourth decade, is the commonest malignancy of the lacrimal gland and accounts for 30% of all epithelial tumours. Other, much rarer, carcinomas include primary adenocarcinoma, muco-epidermoid carcinoma, squamous carcinoma and malignant mixed tumours; malignant mixed tumours arising either within a longstanding pleomorphic adenoma, or within recurrent pleomorphic adenoma after previously incomplete resection.

The diagnosis of lacrimal carcinoma is suggested by an unrelenting, relatively rapid progression of ocular displacement and upper eyelid swelling caused by a non-tender lacrimal gland mass; such patients will often present with a history of less than 6 months (Figure 13.4a). The rapid progression and

pain may suggest acute dacryoadenitis, but failure of any inflammatory lesion of the lacrimal gland to clearly improve within a few weeks should prompt further investigation for malignancy.

CT scan shows expansion of the lacrimal gland by a mass that typically moulds to the globe and extends posteriorly alongside the lateral orbital wall, displacing the lateral rectus medially (Figure 13.4b). In more advanced cases there may be erosive changes in the bone of the lacrimal gland fossa, best shown with bone-window settings. Calcification, usually a few flecks, may be present in up to one-third of malignant lacrimal gland tumours.

The tumour should be biopsied through the upper lid skin crease (Chapter 12). Adenoid cystic carcinoma is composed of solid cords of malignant epithelial cells, often with cystic spaces giving a "Swiss cheese" pattern. The tumour infiltrates well beyond the macroscopic boundaries evident at surgery and on radiological imaging, and adenoid cystic carcinoma has a propensity for perineural spread into the cavernous sinus and pterygo-palatine fossa.

The best method of treatment remains controversial, because recurrences of adenoid cystic carcinoma may be very slowly progressive and can become manifest at more than 10 years after primary treatment; it is likely, therefore, that a "cure" can only be countenanced after 20 years without recurrence. These patients probably do best with removal of the tumor bulk (which can often be almost complete) through an anterior orbitotomy and subsequently they should receive 55–60cGy of radiotherapy to both the orbit and the cavernous sinus (Figure 13.4c). Unless frankly invaded by tumour, the cortical bone of the lateral orbital wall should be left undisturbed as any breach is likely to encourage seeding of tumour cells into the cranial diploe, with a slow and relentless fatal recurrence of local disease (Figure 13.4d). Implantation brachytherapy has been

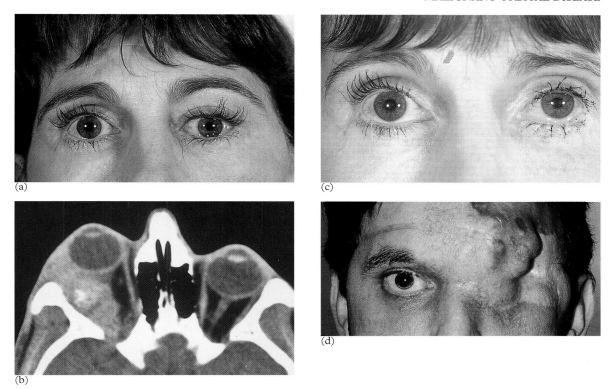

Figure 13.4 (a) A patient with left lacrimal gland carcinoma, (b) such tumours typically producing enlarged lacrimal gland moulding to the globe and extending posteriorly alongside the lateral orbital wall, (c) treatment with debulking and fractionated high-dose radiotherapy to the orbit and cavernous sinus produces good disease control with a satisfactory cosmesis, (d) craniofacial resection may encourage seeding of the tumour into the cranial diploe, with subsequent slow and relentless fatal local recurrence.

advocated as delivering a high radiation dosage to the tumour bed whilst relatively sparing the globe, but it does not, however, treat the cavernous sinus or pterygo-palatine fossa – to which these tumours often extend by perineural invasion.

There is no reliable evidence to suggest that either exenteration or "super-exenteration" (with removal of the neighbouring orbital bones) leads to a reduction of recurrence rate or a prolongation of life; such procedures are associated with a marked disfigurement in relatively young people. Intra-carotid chemotherapy may have a role as an adjunct to radiotherapy in advanced disease.

Dry eye is inevitable with removal of the lacrimal gland and radiotherapy; frequent topical lubricants, together with occlusion of the lacrimal drainage puncta, are often required. Radiation-induced cataract is common at about two years after treatment.

Tumour recurrence occurs relatively late with adenoid cystic carcinoma and the relatively young person may have many years of useful, symptom free life before regrowth of tumour is evident. Unfortunately most patients will eventually suffer a painful and relentlessly progressive local recurrence of the disease (Figure 13.4d), with a high mortality from intracranial recurrence or metastasis.

Other mesenchymal tumours

Sarcomas of the orbit are extremely rare. The highly malignant osteosarcoma is generally secondary to childhood orbital radiotherapy for retinoblastoma; even with radical clearance, the tumour is almost uniformly fatal by two years after diagnosis. Children may present with metastatic Ewing's sarcoma or Wilm's tumour within the orbit and will require systemic therapy after diagnosis.

Fibrosarcoma is a malignant tumour of fibroblasts, which can arise as a primary lesion (Figure 13.5) or as a secondary tumour from adjacent sinuses or at the site of prior radiotherapy. Wide excision, often with exenteration, is recommended and palliation with radiotherapy and chemotherapy may be beneficial. The prognosis for vision and life is variable, but is best for primary juvenile fibrosarcomas.

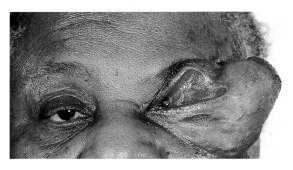

Figure 13.5   Fibrosarcoma recurrence at one year after incomplete tumour resection.

Several rare orbital tumours present with a spectrum of disease, from benign to malignant. Malignant fibrous histiocytoma arises from fascia, muscle or other soft tissues and typically presents as a well-defined mass in the supero-nasal quadrant of the orbit. Recurrence of these radio-resistant and chemo-resistant tumours is common, even after wide excision, and the tumour is associated with a significant mortality. Haemangiopericytoma, likewise, has a spectrum of malignancy and should be treated by wide and, if possible, intact resection.

Leiomyosarcoma, a tumour of smooth muscle, and liposarcomas of various degrees of differentiation have been reported to very rarely involve the orbit.

Orbital lymphoma in adults

Lymphocyte recruiting lesions of the orbit display a spectrum from a benign morphology, showing well-organised follicular pattern (so-called "reactive lymphoid hyperplasia"), through the rare "atypical lymphoid hyperplasia" with poorly organised or disrupted follicular formation, to frank malignant lymphoma. With the advent of histochemical stains specific for various particular types of lymphocytes, their precursors and the follicle dendritic cells, it has become evident in recent years that many lesions labelled "atypical lymphoid hyperplasia" are, in fact, lymphomas displaying various degrees of disorganised follicle formation or destruction.

Orbital lymphomas, about 10% of orbital masses, are almost exclusively non-Hodgkin's B-cell lymphomas, the tumours containing a minority of reactive T lymphocytes and a variable degree of follicular organisation. The few reported T-cell lymphomas involving the orbit are in patients with systemic disease, and advanced Burkitt's lymphoma may spread from the neighbouring sinuses. Dependent on the grade of lymphoma, up to about a half of patients presenting with orbital disease will be found to have systemic involvement within six months of presentation.

Orbital lymphomas present as a slowly progressive, painless subconjunctival "salmon patch" (Figure 13.6) or, if deeper in the orbit, with swelling of the eyelids, globe displacement or diplopia. The typical age of presentation is over 50, although younger individuals may develop the more aggressive, high-grade lymphomas.

CT scan typically shows a moderately well defined soft tissue mass moulding around the globe and affecting – but often not destroying the form of – multiple tissues (such as the lacrimal gland or extraocular muscles) (Figure 13.7); bilateral disease is present in about 25% of cases. Calcification in the lesion and changes in the orbital bones are very unusual, although rarely a longstanding lesion may

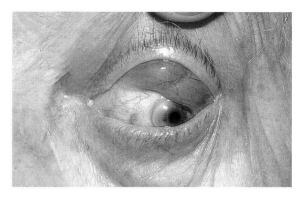

Figure 13.6 Typical "salmon-patch" mass of conjunctival lymphoma.

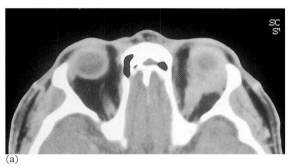

(a)

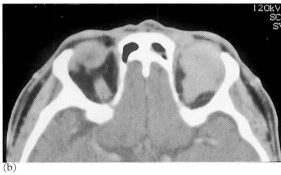

(b)

Figure 13.7 Lymphoma of the lacrimal gland: (a) moulding around the globe and extending into the surrounding fat and (b) levator/superior rectus muscle complex.

expand the neighbouring orbital wall if the bone is thin. Neither the CT nor the MRI characteristics are diagnostic for the condition, being indistinguishable from inflammation, and biopsy is mandatory.

As the contemporary tissue diagnosis and treatment of lymphoproliferative disease is dependent on structural analysis, open biopsy is recommended as it provides a solid piece of tissue with minimal disruption of structure. Fine needle aspiration biopsy will only provide disrupted tissue, with no indication of form. All patients with lymphoid lesions of the orbit should undergo investigation for systemic disease, this including whole-body CT scan and bone-marrow biopsy where the lymphoma is of higher grade (for example, with follicle-centre lymphoma or diffuse large B-cell lymphoma).

Low-grade lymphomas involving the orbit respond well to about 2400cGy fractionated radiotherapy (Figure 13.8), although a slowly progressive lesion in a very frail or moribund patient may be observed. Widespread low-grade systemic disease generally responds well to oral chemotherapy.

Patients with high-grade lymphomas have, however, a much higher chance of systemic

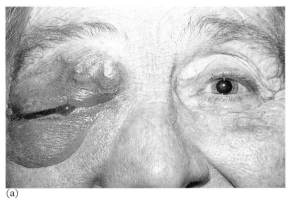

(a)

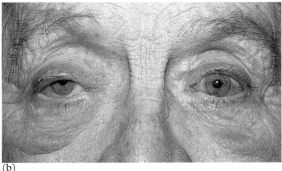

(b)

Figure 13.8 A patient with low-grade orbital and sinus lymphoma, (a) before and (b) at two months after local radiotherapy.

disease and usually require multiple cycles of chemotherapy. If there is significant impairment of orbital function (with, for example, optic neuropathy) then local radiotherapy provides a useful means to accelerate resolution of the orbital disease.

When the disease is confined to the orbit the visual prognosis is excellent and complications are unusual, but the overall mortality is variable. Review for at least 10 years is required, as systemic lymphoma can become evident for many years after the presentation of solely orbital disease.

Method for orbital exenteration

Exenteration, for certain pervasive malignant or benign orbital diseases, involves complete removal of the eyeball, retrobulbar soft tissues and most, or all, of the eyelids. Skin-sparing exenteration provides a very rapid rehabilitation and is particularly useful for benign disease, post-septal intraorbital malignancy and for the palliation of fungating terminal orbital malignancy (Figure 13.9a).

The skin incision should be placed well clear of the malignancy, either near the orbital rim if dealing with extensive eyelid malignancy invading the orbit, or alongside the lash-line if a skin-sparing exenteration; if skin-sparing, the skin and orbicularis oculi muscle should be undermined to the orbital rim. The periosteum is incised just outside the rim, raised intact over the rim and posteriorly into the orbit; resistance to raising the periosteum may be encountered at the arcus marginalis, the trochlear fossa, the interosseous suture lines and the lacrimal crest. It is necessary to cauterise and divide the anterior and posterior ethmoidal vessels in the supero-nasal quadrant, the nasolacrimal duct, and any vessels crossing between the orbit and the lateral orbital wall and floor. Care is required to avoid damage to the lamina papyracea, as entry into the ethmoid sinuses may lead to a chronic sino-orbital fistula.

Once the orbital contents have been mobilised within the periosteum, the posterior tissues are transected about 7–10mm from the apex (Figure 13.9b); this is most readily achieved from the lateral side, using a monopolar diathermy in a blended cutting and coagulation mode. The ophthalmic artery should also be cauterised with bipolar diathermy and any persistent bleeding from the bones should be plugged with bone wax.

With skin-sparing exenteration, the upper ands lower eyelid flaps are sutured together using buried 5/0 absorbable sutures in the orbicularis muscle layer and the skin closed with continuous 6/0 nylon; the aim is to create an air-tight closure to encourage retraction of the socket surface during healing (Figure 13.9c). If a complete exenteration of the eyelids and orbit has been performed, the socket can either be left to granulate or lined with split-thickness skin grafts (Figure 13.9d).

Complications of exenteration include operative leakage of cerebro-spinal fluid, post operative infection, necrosis of flaps and grafts, or delayed socket granulation. Breakdown of the lamina papyracea may lead to communication between the ethmoid sinuses and the exenteration cavity (a sino-orbital fistula) and failure of closure of the nasolacrimal duct may lead to a "blow-hole" fistula.

Secondary orbital tumours

The orbit may be infiltrated by malignant tumours arising in the globe or in any of the surrounding structures, such as the eyelids and paranasal sinuses. If there is extensive orbital involvement, it may be necessary for orbital exenteration as part of the surgical rehabilitation.

Eyelid tumours

Tumours originating in the lids, particularly meibomian gland carcinoma and neglected basal cell or squamous carcinomas, can spread

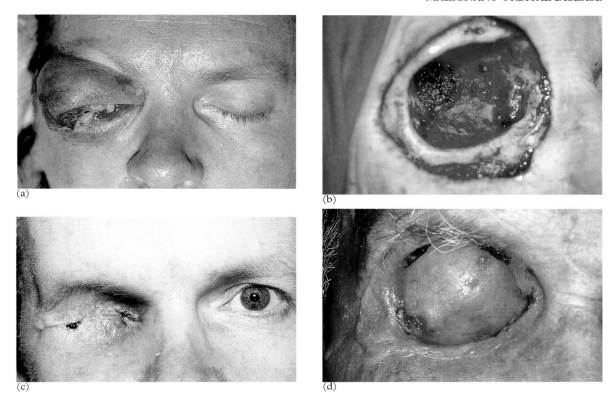

Figure 13.9 (a) Fungating melanoma in young patient with terminal disease, (b) the periosteum is incised outside the orbital rim, separated from the orbital walls, the orbital contents are removed leaving a 7–10mm stump at the orbital apex, to prevent CSF leakage, (c) with skin-sparing exenteration there is a rapid healing and retraction of the skin over a few weeks after surgery; (d) where the eyelid skin has been excised, the socket can either be left to heal by granulation, or else grafted with split-thickness skin.

posteriorly through the septal connective tissue to enter the orbit. Diplopia on extreme gaze is an important early sign suggesting orbital invasion and fixation of the mass to the underlying bone suggests more advanced disease.

Perineural invasion, usually along branches of the frontal nerve and liable to cause pain, is commonest with squamous cell carcinoma and may occur with primary tumours arising above the brow line and without clear clinical signs of a mass causing orbital invasion. Sebaceous (meibomian gland) carcinoma has a propensity for intraepithelial pagetoid spread within the conjunctiva and skin and an apparently localised eyelid mass may actually widely involve the surface of the globe and eyelids, in some cases necessitating exenteration.

Tumours of the paranasal sinuses

The commonest epithelial tumour to secondarily involve the orbit by direct invasion is squamous carcinoma arising in the paranasal sinuses or pharynx; extension can rarely occur without bone erosion, but by perineural spread through, for example, the ethmoid foramina or the inferior orbital fissure. Orbital involvement represents advanced disease and the prognosis is usually poor. Management often involves diagnostic biopsy and later wide surgical clearance (including exenteration if there is direct orbital involvement) with radiotherapy.

Other paranasal tumours that may involve the orbit by direct invasion are adenoid cystic carcinoma, adenocarcinoma, esthesioneuroblastoma and melanoma.

Tumours of intraocular origin

Uveal malignant melanoma is the most common primary intraocular tumour in adults and may spread directly to the orbit through the emissary veins. More rarely, aggressive tumours may reach the orbit by direct scleral invasion or through the optic nerve head. To date, patients with orbital extension of uveal melanoma have a very poor prognosis as there is frequently systemic disease; future advances in tumour-directed chemotherapy may, however, improve the outlook for this situation.

Extraocular extension of retinoblastoma (the commonest intraocular malignancy in childhood) occurs in approximately 8% of patients, but can present later in life as a lump in an anophthalmic socket. After enucleation of the eyes with extrascleral extension of retinoblastoma, adjuvant treatment often combines systemic chemotherapy with orbital radiotherapy, although the prognosis is relatively poor.

Adult metastatic orbital disease

Although in adults systemic tumours will metastasise more commonly to the uveal tract, orbital metastases represent 2–3% of all orbital tumours and occasionally will be the first manifestation of an occult primary tumour. In children, however, distant tumours most frequently metastasise to the orbit. As the orbit does not contain any lymphatic channels, it is presumed that haematological spread is responsible for metastatic disease.

In adults the commonest primary sites are breast, prostate, lung, kidney and gastrointestinal tract and they may present with painful proptosis and diplopia, such that a misdiagnosis of orbital inflammation or abscess may be made (Figure 13.10). It is important that the possibility of orbital malignancy is considered, and open biopsy undertaken, whenever a disease progresses despite treatment.

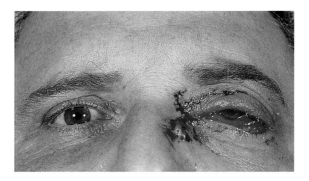

Figure 13.10 Patient referred after exploration for presumed orbital abscess; subsequent biopsy of the inferior rectus muscle demonstrated necrosis of a metastatic carcinoma.

The mainstay of therapy is local treatment with 55–60cGy fractionated radiotherapy, although in some cases there may be a role for surgical debulking prior to radiotherapy. Patients with a solitary orbital metastasis from a carcinoid or renal adenocarcinoma should be considered for exenteration.

The prognosis is variable, but generally the main goal of treatment is palliative with avoidance of discomfort and preservation of vision if possible. Dry eye is a major problem after the high dosage of radiation required for treatment of malignancy.

Rare primary malignant orbital tumours of adulthood

Malignant neurilemmoma, extremely rare and of Schwann cell origin, may arise *de novo* or in association with neurofibromatosis. It presents as a slowly progressive lid mass or proptosis and CT scan shows an ill-defined mass with possible destruction of adjacent bone. Management involves wide surgical clearance, often requiring orbital exenteration, and adjunctive radiotherapy or chemotherapy. The prognosis is poor as these malignant tumours tend to spread from the orbit into the middle cranial fossa and metastasise to the lungs.

Orbital haemangiopericytoma is a tumour that has a spectrum of invasiveness, from well-circumscribed, benign disease to infiltrative malignancy. Treatment of the benign lesions is intact excision, which is curative, whereas the malignant variants require wide clearance, usually by orbital exenteration. Local and remote recurrence are fairly common with malignant haemangiopericytoma.

Further reading

Affeldt JC, Minchler DS, Azen SP, Yeh L. Prognosis in uveal melanoma with uveal extension. *Arch Ophthalmol* 1980; **98**:1975–9.

Bartley GB, Garrity JA, Waller RR *et al*. Orbital exenteration at the Mayo clinic. 1967-1986. *Ophthalmology* 1989; **96**:468–73.

Ferry AP, Font RL. Carcinoma metastatic to the eye and orbit. A clinicopathologic study of 227 cases. *Arch Ophthalmol* 1974; **92**:276–86.

Fratkin JD, Shammas HF, Miller SD. Disseminated Hodgkin's disease with orbital involvement. *Arch Ophthalmol* 1978; **96**:102–4.

Goldberg RA, Rootman J, Cline RA. Tumours metastatic to the orbit: a changing clinical picture. *Surv Ophthalmol* 1990; **35**:1–24.

Mamalis N, Grey AM, Good JS, McLeish WM, Anderson RL. Embryonal rhabdomyosarcoma of the orbit in a 35-year-old man. *Ophthalmic Surgery* 1994; **25**:332–5.

Meekins B, Dutton JJ, Proia AD. Primary orbital leiomyosarcoma: a case report and review of the literature. *Arch Ophthalmol* 1988; **106**:82–6.

Rose GE, Wright JE. Exenteration for benign orbital disease. *Br J Ophthalmol* 1994; **78**:14–18.

Rose GE, Wright JE. Pleomorphic adenomas of the lacrimal gland. *Br J Ophthalmol* 1992; **76**:395–400.

Schworm HD, Boergen KP, Stefain FH. The initial clinical manifestations of rhabdomyosarcoma. *Ophthalmology* 1995; **92**:362–5.

Shields CL, Sheilds JA, Peggs M. Metastatic tumours of the orbit. *Ophthal Plast Reconstr Surg* 1988; **4**:73–80.

Sohaib SA, Moseley I, Wright JE. Orbital rhabdomyosarcoma – the radiological characteristics. *Clin Radiol* 1998; **53**:357–62.

Weber AL, Jakobiec FA, Sabates NR. Lymphoproliferative disease of the orbit. *Neuroimaging Clin N Am* 1996; **1**:93–111.

Wright JE, Rose GE, Garner A. Primary malignant neoplasms of the lacrimal gland. *Br J Ophthalmol* 1992; **76**:401–7.

14 Orbital trauma

Brett O'Donnell

Eye injuries are a common accompaniment to major orbital trauma and an immediate assessment of the eye is essential, but may be difficult due to eyelid swelling and bruising. If the lids can be opened by sustained traction without pressure on the globe, an effort should be made to ascertain the visual acuity, the presence of a relative afferent papillary defect, the state and reaction of the pupil, and the state of the globe. Although the intraocular pressure is likely to be spuriously elevated due to both swollen orbital tissues and eyelid manipulation, a very low pressure should alert the clinician to the possibility of a rupture of the globe.

The presence of enophthalmos or exophthalmos should be noted, although traumatic enophthalmos may not be manifest for several weeks until the post-traumatic oedema and bruising has settled. Proptosis usually indicates significant injury to retrobulbar tissues and may be accompanied by a global reduction in eye movements, these ocular ductions not improving until several weeks after injury.

A neurological examination, with especial reference to the first six cranial nerves, should be performed and the presence of a palsy of eye movements (third, fourth or sixth cranial nerves) may indicate an epidural or subdural haematoma, fractures in the region of the sphenoid or orbital apex, direct trauma to the motor nerves, or an intra-orbital haemorrhage causing a compressive neuropathy. Examination of the trigeminal (fifth cranial) nerve should include assessment of sensation to the forehead, cheek, nose, gums and cornea.

Fractures of the orbital floor and medial wall

The indirect, "blowout" fracture of the orbital floor occurs when a major blunt blow is applied across the anterior orbital entrance, the fracture resulting from hydraulic collapse of the orbital floor and possibly by transmission of energy from a transient deformation of the inferior orbital rim. Typically one edge of the fracture involves the infraorbital nerve canal and a transient neuropraxia of this nerve is extremely common, with hypoaesthesia of the ipsilateral cheek, side of nose and upper gum.

Unlike most direct fractures of the orbital floor, the blowout fracture occurs without breach of the orbital rim. The rise in orbital pressure during the blow causes a herniation of orbital tissues through the floor defect, the extremes being either a large prolapse of tissues through an extensive bone defect or a "pinch" of tissues through a tiny crack in the floor. Direct entrapment of the inferior rectus in the fracture line is extremely rare, but diplopia probably results from a combination of contusion of orbital tissues and from entrapment of the fascial planes around inferior rectus muscle.

Comminuted blowout fractures of the medial orbital wall can occur in isolation, but are generally part of an orbital floor blowout fracture. Orbital emphysema, usually the result of nose-blowing, is commoner with ethmoid fractures and the ophthalmic circulation may be embarrassed if the entrapped air causes an undue rise in the orbital pressures; this ophthalmic emergency should be treated urgently by aspiration of air or incision and drainage of the orbital spaces, or an irreversible loss of vision may result. Direct medial wall fractures from blunt trauma also involve the nasal bones, the lacrimal bone and the frontal process of the maxilla, being commonly manifest as a depressed nasal bridge and telecanthus.

Assessment

Any patient with major orbital trauma is likely to have a fracture of the orbital wall or ocular injury. Specific features suggestive of blowout fracture include vertical diplopia with restriction of up or down gaze, pain on extremes of eye movement, hypoaesthesia in the infraorbital nerve territory, periocular emphysema, or enophthalmos and hypoglobus. Forced duction testing will confirm that the restriction of eye movement is of mechanical origin.

Unless there is marked dental artefact, direct coronal CT scans at a bone-imaging window are the investigation of choice (Figure 14.1); not only is the orbital floor better shown than that after reformatting of axial scans, but the orbital apex and the other orbital walls are also well shown.

Most orbital floor blowout fractures do not require surgery and eye movements will often return to normal over several weeks to months. Orthoptics assessment, with sequential Hess charts and fields of binocular single vision, is useful for following the course of recovery and detecting those who are unlikely to return to normal ocular balance.

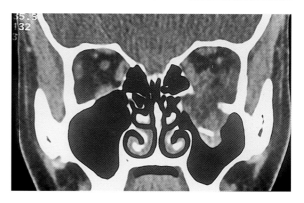

Figure 14.1 Coronal CT scan showing blowout fracture of the medial part of the orbital floor and inferior part of the ethmoid lamina papyracea.

Typically the small, linear fracture causes the greatest disturbance of ocular motility, whereas large fractures with comminution of the orbital floor tend to recover full eye movements. Persistent diplopia within 30° of the primary position is the main indication for surgery and, for most, diplopia on down-gaze is particularly troublesome as it interferes with reading and negotiating stairs. Certain occupations, however, demand frequent use of up-gaze as, for example, with decorators, plasterers, certain sportsmen and pilots.

Cosmetically evident if greater than about 2mm, this degree of enophthalmos generally indicates a significant displacement of bone that merits orbital wall repair. Enophthalmos may not be evident for many weeks until post-traumatic orbital oedema has settled but, if manifest is early, it suggests a major fracture justifying early intervention at 7–14 days after injury – when much of the acute haemorrhage and oedema has settled, but before fibrosis has occurred.

Apart from the presence of marked enophthalmos that justifies early intervention, the timing of surgery remains controversial. There is no good evidence that recovery of ocular motility is improved by early surgery, although the gross restriction of movement due to fascial entrapment in hairline fractures

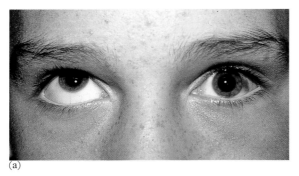

(a)

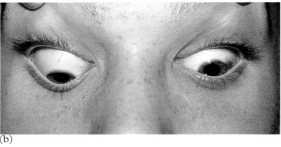

(b)

Figure 14.2   Gross restriction of up (a) and down (b) gaze after a "hairline" blowout fracture of the orbital floor with entrapment of fascia around inferior retus muscle.

(Figure 14.2) may recover better with the release of entrapped tissues within a day or two of injury.

Management

The assessment and treatment of systemic, facial and cranial injury takes precedence over the repair of orbital fractures. The patient with acute orbital fracture involving the paranasal sinuses should be instructed not to blow his/her nose for 10 days and, in view of the sight-threatening nature of acute orbital cellulitis, a short course of systemic antibiotics should be considered. Oral anti-inflammatory medications may be given after injury to accelerate the resolution of orbital inflammation and oedema.

Orbital floor repair

If surgical repair is indicated, then the orbital floor is readily approached through a lower eyelid swinging flap (Chapter 11) or a subciliary skin-muscle blepharoplasty flap (Chapter 8). Using one of these routes, the orbital rim is exposed and the periosteum incised about 5mm outside the rim, to leave a margin of periosteum for adequate closure in front of any orbital floor implant. The periosteum is raised into the orbit, across the orbital floor until the site of fracture is located and then the periosteum around the sides of the fracture site is raised to define the extent of tissue incarceration; particular care must be taken laterally, as this area is liable to major haemorrhage from the infraorbital neurovascular bundle in the area of the inferior orbital fissure. There should be a clinically evident improvement in the forced duction test after the incarcerated orbital tissues are released completely from the fracture site and the whole of the fracture edge should be visible; typically there is a ledge of normal orbital floor at the posterior edge of the fracture site. Although often not possible, the sinus mucosa should be kept intact to avoid formation of sino-orbital fistula.

Once the orbital contents have been completely freed from the fracture site, an implant may be shaped and positioned across the defect in the orbital floor and medial wall (Figure 14.3). Where the repair is for release of entrapped tissues (rather than volume enhancement), it is essential to place the rear of the implant on the intact fragment of orbital floor at the orbital apex, behind the point of emergence of the infraorbital nerve from the inferior orbital fissure. Bulky implants should be avoided within 1cm of the orbital apex, as thick materials may bear upon the optic nerve or ophthalmic artery and lead to blindness, and any materials should be inserted gently and not forced into place. Likewise, when placing the material it is very important to avoid snagging of the orbital fat with the back edge of the implant, or motility disorders will result. The most useful implant materials include porous polyethylene and silicone sheeting, although silicone is

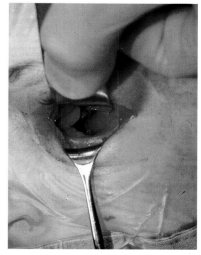

(a)

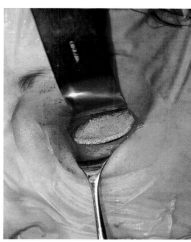

(b)

Figure 14.3 Implant material placed across an orbital floor fracture, approached through a lower eyelid swinging flap: (a) orbital floor pre- and (b) post insertion of implant.

inadvisable where there has been a breach of sinus mucosa; whilst still widely used, bone grafts have the disadvantage of reabsorption and donor-site morbidity. Microplate fixation may be necessary where there has been extensive damage to the orbital walls or fracture of the orbital rim, although treatment of such facial fractures is outside the realm of the ophthalmic surgeon.

The anterior edge of the orbital periosteum is closed with a 5/0 absorbable suture, the lower eyelid approach repaired in layers with a 6/0 absorbable suture and the eyelid placed on upward traction with a 4/0 nylon suture. The site is padded with a firm elastic dressing.

Fractures of the medial orbital wall can be readily repaired during orbital floor repair, with extension of the flexible implant upwards alongside the medial defect. For isolated fractures of the medial wall, however, it is possible to use either the extended post-caruncular incision, directed postero-medially onto the orbital wall, or the aesthetically less desirable Lynch incision, through the skin of the nasal part of the upper eyelid and medial to the inner canthus.

The patient should be nursed head-up after surgery and it is important that any severe or increasing pain is reported. Where pain is severe or increasing, the vision in the affected eye and the state of the orbit should be checked; a very tense orbit with markedly decreased vision, a relative afferent pupillary defect and loss of eye movements, suggests accumulation of orbital haemorrhage and this may lead to irreversible visual loss. If this emergency appears to be developing, the operative site should be reopened at the "bedside", without delay, and any accumulation of blood allowed to drain.

The patient should refrain from nose blowing for 10 days after orbital floor repair and should be prescribed a course of systemic antibiotics and anti-inflammatory medications. It is possible that eye movement exercises performed several times daily, with forced ductions to the extremes of range, may increase the recovery of tissue compliance and speed the resolution of post operative diplopia; if, however, diplopia persists at several months after repair then squint surgery may be of value when the Hess charts are stable.

Complications

Post operative haemorrhage, with threat to vision, is the most feared complication and should be recognised and treated promptly.

The risk of this major complication may be reduced by recognition of the various arterial branches that cross between the orbit and the walls (the branches to the infraorbital nerve and the anterior ethmoidal vessels being the most troublesome in this context) and appropriate coagulation of the vessels.

Increased infraorbital nerve hypoaesthesia is fairly common and generally recovers. Transient alteration in muscle balance is almost inevitable, this typically settling over a week or two, but capture of the released orbital tissues by an edge of the implant should be avoided as it may permanently worsen motility.

Infection, more common with entrance into the sinus cavity, may occur soon after surgery (Figure 14.4) and necessitates removal of the implant with later repair after the infection has settled on systemic therapy. Late infection may occur where maxillary sinusitis spreads through a thin interface into the site of orbital repair.

Migration of the implant is less common with integrating implants, such as porous polyethylene, and frank extrusion from the operative site (Figure 14.5) is almost unknown with avoidance of direct incision over the inferior orbital rim – an unsightly surgical approach used widely in the past. Formation of a pneumatocoele around non-integrating implants such as silicone (Figure 14.6), lined by respiratory epithelium that has migrated through an sino-orbital fistula, may be avoided

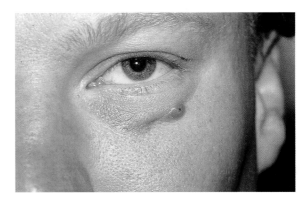

Figure 14.5   Late extrusion of a silicone implant through a direct incision over the orbital rim.

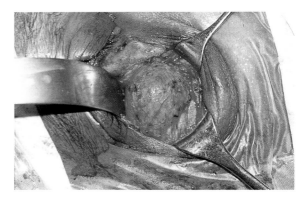

Figure 14.6   Air-filled cavity (in communication with the maxillary sinus) that has formed around a silicone sheet implant for repair of an orbital fracture.

by using integrating implants where there is a defect into the sinuses at the time of surgery; where a pneumatocoele forms, it can later be excised and the defect repaired, if necessary, with an integrating implant material.

Surgical approaches through the lower eyelid may rarely lead to a cicatricial retraction of the lower lid, with secondary entropion or ectropion.

Damage to the lacrimal drainage system, either during exposure of a fracture site or due to bearing of the implant on the nasolacrimal duct, may lead to epiphora that may require dacryocystorhinostomy. Likewise, surgery on the medial orbital wall carries a very minor risk of cerebro-spinal fluid leak or intracranial damage.

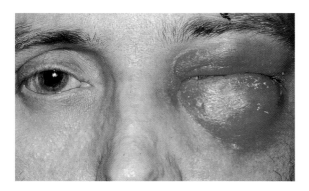

Figure 14.4   Patient referred with acute infection of an orbital floor implant.

Fractures of the orbital roof, zygoma and mid-face

Fractures of the orbital roof are uncommon and usually accompany major head injury, larger fractures often being comminuted and involving the frontal sinuses, the cribriform plate or intracranial injury; the ophthalmologist is, therefore, unlikely to be in charge of the primary management of these cases. Similarly, midfacial fractures are treated by maxillo–facial surgeons and the ophthalmologist's role is in the assessment of visual function, treatment of the ocular injury and in the late management of associated soft tissue injury and diplopia.

Assessment

Orbital roof injury should be suspected where head trauma is accompanied by a large upper eyelid haematoma, hypoglobus, restricted up gaze and sensory loss over the forehead (Figure 14.7). Late manifestations include deformity of the orbital rim underlying the brow and failure of descent of the upper eyelid during down gaze due to adhesions between the fracture site and the levator muscle.

Tripod fracture of the zygoma, with disarticulation from the neighbouring frontal bone and maxilla, tends to occur with a major blow to the cheek and is manifest by a flattening of the prominence of the cheek (although this may be masked by overlying haematoma), by palpable discontinuity of the orbital rim, by tenderness with upward pressure below the zygomatic arch, and by an ipsilateral buccal haematoma.

Le Fort fractures involve the maxilla and extend posteriorly through the pterygoid plates. The orbit is involved in types II and III Le Fort fractures, both extending across the medial part of the orbit at the level of the cribriform plate, but the type II fracture (the commonest) passes infero-laterally to the level of the inferior orbital fissure, whereas the type III fracture extends laterally higher in the orbit, through the zygomatico-temporal suture line. It is unlikely that the ophthalmologist will be required to identify such fractures, which are characterised by dental malocclusion.

When one of these fractures is identified, adequate CT imaging should be performed to include an area clear of the clinical site of injury; damage at the optic canal should be identified prior to surgery, with particular care being taken to avoid damage to the nerve or its circulation by disturbance of bone fragments near the orbital apex or canal. Treatment of these fractures is by open reduction, microplate fixation and dental stabilisation.

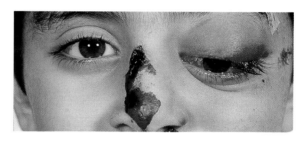

Figure 14.7 Child presenting with a delayed onset of severe compressive optic neuropathy due to a large subperiosteal haematoma along the orbital roof; the child had sustained a blunt orbital injury a week before, with fracture of the orbital roof.

Management

Small fractures of the orbital roof are managed conservatively if they cause no functional deficit and only minimal irregularity of the orbital rim and brow. Small bone fragments that interfere with the function of the levator or superior rectus muscles should be repositioned or removed, either through the open wound at the time of primary repair, or through an incision in the upper eyelid skin crease. Larger bone fragments require reduction and microplate fixation, although most such surgery is beyond the realm of the ophthalmic surgeon and involves a multi-disciplinary approach.

Adherence of the levator muscle or upper eyelid scars to fractures of the orbital rim or roof may cause lagophthalmos and exposure keratitis. This may be treated by exploration of the orbital roof through an upper eyelid incision, division of any adhesions and placement of a dermis-fat graft sutured inside the orbital rim, to the periosteum of the orbital roof.

Complications

Both the injury itself and the surgery for the repair of these complex fractures may be associated with supraorbital nerve injury, loss of other ocular motor innervation due to damage near the superior orbital fissure, orbital emphysema and pneumocephalus, a subperiosteal haematoma with a secondary compressive optic neuropathy (Figure 14.7) and associated intracranial injuries. Late complications include persistent ptosis, due either to mechanical damage or denervation, lagophthalmos due to scarring and retraction of the upper eyelid or levator muscle and chronic or recurrent sinusitis, particularly that of the frontal sinus.

Intraorbital foreign bodies

The site of entry of an orbital foreign body may be self-sealing and easily overlooked. High-speed foreign bodies are more likely to penetrate the globe, whereas low-speed ones (such as twigs) are more likely to spare the globe. Failure to remove an unsterile foreign body is likely to result in an intraorbital or intracranial abscess, or an externally draining sinus (Figure 14.8).

The prime investigation for localisation is thin-slice axial and direct coronal CT scan (Figure 14.9) and MRI should be considered – but only after excluding the presence of intraorbital ferro-magnetic materials – where wood and other materials of vegetable origin are thought to be present.

Treatment

Removal of an orbital foreign body is indicated when there is thought to be

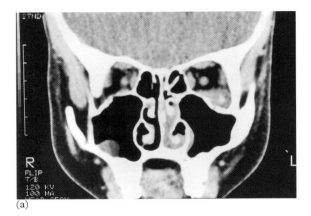

(a)

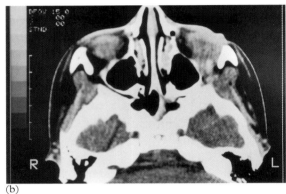

(b)

Figure 14.8 Wooden foreign body in the inferior part of the orbit and the pterygopalatine fossa: (a) coronal and (b) axial view.

reversible visual impairment, persistent pain, diplopia, inflammation or infection, or when the object is palpable in the anterior part of the orbit. Unless the foreign body is visible under the conjunctiva, surgery should be under general anaesthesia as location of the materials can be difficult. When a foreign body is inert and posterior within the orbit (Figure 14.10), it can be left in place and the risk of surgical damage to the orbital contents avoided.

All organic matter must be removed, as this typically incites a vigorous inflammatory response and is liable to infection. Non-metallic inorganic materials, such as glass, stone or plastics, may generally be left and observed and non-reactive metals, such as stainless steel, steel or aluminium, are well tolerated. Copper-containing metals, including

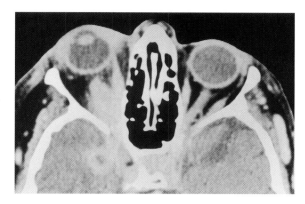

Figure 14.9 Inferior orbital foreign body with associated brain abscess.

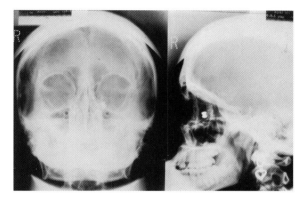

Figure 14.10 Airgun pellet deep within orbit, thus not requiring removal.

brass, should be removed as they cause marked suppurative inflammation. Intraorbital lead can be left, as it does not appear to cause systemic toxicity and intraorbital iron does not have the toxicity of intraocular iron.

Injury to orbital soft tissues

Damage to extraocular muscles

Avulsion of extraocular muscles is rare and usually results from a penetrating orbital injury with a "hooking" force, seen occasionally with deliberate attempts at enucleation during assault (Figure 14.11). CT scan allows an assessment of the state of the musculature, although repair is often difficult

due to oedema, haemorrhage and retraction of the muscle into the orbit. When enucleation has been achieved, orbital oedema may be extreme and bacterial contamination likely; in these circumstances primary implantation of a ball is likely to fail and this should be deferred until both the oedema and the risk of infection has settled.

Explosive injuries result in ragged wounds with widespread intraorbital debris, and should be treated by extensive cleaning of tissues, debridement where necessary and repair of the globe and eyelids where possible. Where there has been a major loss of eyelid tissues, the principles of reconstruction are similar to those for eyelid repair after excision of tumours (Chapter 5), although this may need to be deferred until the acute oedema has improved; whilst awaiting reconstruction, the repaired globe should be kept moist with regular lubricant/antibiotic ointments and a "moisture chamber" such as, for example, a cling-film application over a Cartella shield.

Optic nerve injury

Injury to the optic nerve can either be direct, due to penetrating orbital foreign bodies or avulsion, or indirect as part of a major head injury, with fractures around the orbital apex – where bone fragments may impinge on the nerve – or actually involving the optic canal.

Optic nerve damage anterior to the entrance of the central retinal artery causes visual loss with retinal artery occlusion, whereas optic nerve avulsion (Figure 14.11) produces extensive peripapillary haemorrhage and a later fibroglial reaction.

The commonest site for injury to the posterior part of the optic nerve is in the bony canal (Figure 14.12) and, more rarely, in the intracranial nerve or chiasm. Optic neuropathy may occur with or without fracture of the canal and recent CT studies suggest that sphenoid fractures are more common than previously

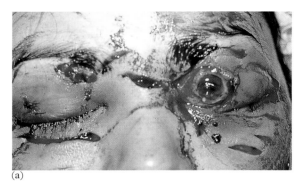

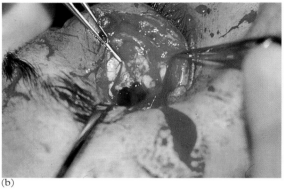

Figure 14.11 (a) Major avulsion of the globes and eyelids during assault with a claw-hammer, (b) the scleral defect is evident at the site of optic nerve avulsion.

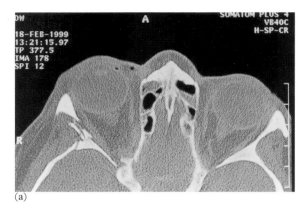

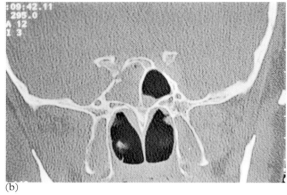

Figure 14.12 Fracture of the right optic nerve canal with severe optic neuropathy.

thought. It is believed that the energy of impact and shearing forces due to deceleration are transmitted to the area of the optic canal, resulting in axonal damage and tearing of the pial vessels supplying the intracanalicular optic nerve; oedema of the injured tissues and post-traumatic vasospasm will both exacerbate neural ischaemic damage and this forms a rational basis for the use of high-dose corticosteroids after such injuries. The role of optic canal decompression, however, remains in doubt.

Treatment of indirect optic neuropathy may be empirically based on the results for spinal cord injury: a loading dosage of 30mg/kg Methyl-prednisolone within 8 hours of injury is followed by an infusion of about 5mg/kg/hr for 24 hours after injury. A tailing dosage of prednisolone or dexamethasone may then be continued for a few days.

Surgery may be considered for removal of bone fragments, where these are thought to be causing a compressive optic neuropathy, and for drainage of intraorbital haematomas. Although visual improvement has been reported after drainage of haematomas from within the optic nerve sheath, there is no evidence that this procedure actually alters the natural course of the condition.

Decompression of the optic canal, by removal of the lateral wall of the sphenoid sinus where it overlies the optic canal, has not been shown to improve visual recovery after injury to the intracanalicular optic nerve; it may, however, have a role where vision deteriorates in the face of adequate medical therapy. Decompression may be achieved through a trans-cranial or a trans-ethmoidectomy approach and may be usefully incorporated as part of an open repair of cranio-facial injuries. Because of the proximity of the internal carotid artery to the operative site, an otorhinolaryngologist or neurosurgeon familiar with the regional anatomy best performs the procedure.

Subperiosteal haematoma

A subperiosteal haematoma of the orbit may follow blunt trauma, is usually superiorly within the orbit and the presentation – with a slowly progressive displacement of the globe – may lead to delayed diagnosis (Figure 14.7). The haematoma should be drained through a transcutaneous approach and a vacuum drain left in place until the bleeding settles; compressive optic neuropathy, whilst rare, dictates urgent intervention.

Surgical trauma to the orbit

The orbital contents may occasionally be damaged due to inadvertent entry into the orbit during endoscopic sinus surgery and may result in devastating complications, such as severe motility restriction or blindness (Figure 14.13). Direct damage to the orbital fat, muscles and, more rarely, optic nerve, may occur, especially during power-assisted debridement of diseased sinus tissues. The most important point in the management of inadvertent orbital entry is recognition and immediate cessation of further surgery; in particular the orbit should be observed for signs of traction on the orbital tissues and for small movements of the globe.

Injury to the ethmoidal arteries may result in orbital haemorrhage with compressive optic neuropathy and this may require anterior orbitotomy, drainage of the haematoma and diathermy of damaged vessels.

Orbital haemorrhage more commonly follows orbital surgery or after retrobulbar or peribulbar injections for intraocular and periocular surgery; it may also occur with blepharoplasty, when it is thought to arise from

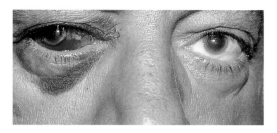

Figure 14.13 Blindness and gross right exotropia after avulsion of the right medial rectus, inferior oblique and optic nerve during endoscopic sinus surgery.

traction damage to small deep orbital vessels. A venous bleed is of slower onset and will usually self tamponade with vision frequently recovering. Firm orbital pressure may assist tamponade and a lateral cantholysis after 5–10 minutes may assist reduction in intraorbital pressure after tamponade has occurred.

A rapid development of proptosis is likely to be arterial bleeding and should be dealt with by very firm orbital pressure applied for about 8–10 minutes, but being released for about 15 seconds every 2 minutes to allow ocular perfusion. If the orbital pressure rises to a very high level, with loss of eye movements and vision not attributable to local anaesthesia, then the orbit should be drained through a skin incision in the affected quadrant; once the skin is opened, a closed pair of blunt-ended scissors should be gently advanced about 3cm into the orbital fat of the affected quadrant and the blades gently opened to spread the tissues and encourage drainage of blood and tissue fluid. This manoeuvre is generally sufficient to release the orbital tamponade, with restoration of vision, and a drain should be placed until the bleeding has stopped.

Further reading

Anderson RL, Panje WR, Gross CE. Optic nerve blindness following blunt forehead trauma. *Ophthalmology* 1982; **89**:445–55.

Baker RS, Epstein AD. Ocular motor abnormalities from head trauma. *Surv Ophthalmol* 1991; **35**:245–67.

Biesman BS, Hornblass A, Lisman R, Kazlas M. Diplopia after surgical repair of orbital floor fractures. *Ophthal Plast Reconstr Surg* 1996; **1**:9–16.

Bracken MB, Shepard MJ, Collins WF *et al.* A randomised, controlled trial of methyl prednisolone or naloxone in the treatment of acute spinal cord injury. Results of the Second National Acute Spinal Cord Injury Study. *N Eng J Med* 1990; **322**:1405–11.

Crompton MR. Visual lesions in closed head injury. *Brain* 1970; **93**:785–92.

Dutton JJ. Management of blowout fractures of the orbital floor. Editorial. *Surv Ophthalmol* 1990; **35**:279–80.

Goldberg RA, Marmor MF, Shorr N, Christenbury JD. Blindness following blepharoplasty: two case reports, and a discussion of management. *Ophthalmic Surg* 1990; **21**:85–9.

Goldberg RA, Steinsapir KD. Extracranial optic canal decompression: indications and technique. *Ophthal Plast Reconstr Surg* 1996; **12**:163–70.

Gross CE, DeKock JR, Panje WR, *et al.* Evidence for orbital deformation that may contribute to monocular blindness following minor frontal head trauma. *J Neurosurg* 1998; **55**:963–6.

Guy J, Sherwood M, Day AL. Surgical treatment of progressive visual loss in traumatic optic neuropathy. Report of two cases. *J Neurosurg* 1989; **70**;799–801.

Harris GJ, Garcia GH, Logani SC, Murphy ML. Correlation of preoperative computed tomography and post operative ocular motility in orbital blowout fractures. *Ophthal Plast Reconstr Surg* 2000; **16**:179–87.

Rose GE, Collin JRO. Dermofat grafts to the extraconal orbital space. *Br J Ophthalmol* 1992; **76**:408–11.

Smith B, Regan WF Jr. Blowout fracture of the orbit: mechanism and correction of internal orbital fractures. *Am J Ophthalmol* 1957; **44**:733–9.

Steinsapir KD, Goldberg RA. Traumatic optic neuropathy. *Surv Ophthalmol* 1994; **38**:487–518.

Streitman MJ, Otto RA, Sakal CS. Anatomic considerations in complications of endoscopic and intranasal sinus surgery. *Ann Otol Rhinol Laryngol* 1994; **103**:105–9.

15 Basic external lacrimal surgery

Cornelius René

Watering eyes result from excessive tear production (hypersecretion), reduced drainage or a combination of the two. A good history and thorough assessment (Chapter 10) are essential to determine the nature of the underlying problem and decide on its management.

Dacryocystorhinostomy indications

Dacryocystorhinostomy (DCR) involves removal of the bone lying between the lacrimal sac and the nose, with anastomosis between the lacrimal sac and nasal mucosa; the lacrimal sac, with the internal opening of the common canaliculus, is incorporated into the lateral wall of the nose and provides a direct route for tears to reach the nose.

The usual indication for DCR is complete or partial obstruction of the nasolacrimal duct: such obstruction can cause skin excoriation, visual impairment, social embarrassment, chronic ocular discharge and acute or chronic dacryocystitis. Less common indications for DCR include lacrimal calculi, facial nerve palsy, gustatory lacrimation (crocodile tears), and lacrimal sac trauma. In the presence of lacrimal sac mucocoele, DCR is mandatory prior to intraocular surgery because of the risk of post operative endophthalmitis.

Patients with acute dacryocystitis require treatment with systemic antibiotics prior to undertaking DCR.

Anaesthesia

Open lacrimal surgery can be performed under general or local anaesthesia. Local anaesthesia with sedation provides excellent intraoperative haemostasis, but may be associated with somewhat prolonged post operative nasal oozing. Some patients and surgeons, however, prefer general anaesthesia with controlled intraoperative hypotension; with newer short-acting anaesthetic drugs, daycase surgery under general anaesthesia is readily achievable in most cases.

Local anaesthesia is particularly useful for elderly or debilitated patients who are unfit for general anaesthesia. The anterior nasal space is sprayed with 4% lignocaine and packed with 1·2m of 12·5mm ribbon gauze thoroughly moistened with 2ml of a 10% cocaine solution, this producing very effective intranasal anaesthesia and mucosal vasoconstriction. Using angled nasal forceps, short loops of the ribbon gauze are firmly packed far anteriorly and superiorly within the nasal space – high against the lateral wall of the nose and the anterior aspect of the middle turbinate, at the site of the proposed rhinostomy. Although not essential, the headlight and nasal speculum may aid correct placement of the nasal pack. A regional block of the anterior ethmoidal branch of the nasociliary nerve is given by infiltration of 2–3ml of 0·5% bupivacaine with 1:200,000 adrenaline along the medial wall of the orbit, immediately above the medial canthal tendon and below the trochlea. Additional anaesthesia and vasoconstriction at the site of incision is achieved by skin infiltration with 2–3ml of the same local anaesthetic preparation. To achieve maximal vasoconstriction, the local anaesthetic should be administered at least 10 minutes before surgery commences and may usefully be given just prior to scrubbing, skin preparation and sterile draping; topical ocular anaesthesia, such as 0.5% amethocaine eyedrops, is also required at the time of surgery.

Vasoconstriction and haemostasis

During local anaesthesia, nasal packing with cocaine generally provides sufficient vasoconstriction of the nasal mucosa, although during surgery it can be supplemented by the intramucosal or submucosal injection of a local anaesthetic (such as 2% lidocaine) with 1:200,000 adrenaline. With this technique, intraoperative bleeding tends to be minimal and any oozing into the nasal space may be readily aspirated with a 12G bronchial aspiration catheter placed within the mid-nasal space throughout the procedure. Where general anaesthesia is used, vasoconstriction of the nasal mucosa is equally important and, after preparation of the sterile field, is most conveniently achieved by placing three cotton-tipped applicators, moistened with 1:1000 adrenaline, high in the antero-superior nasal space. Infiltration of local anaesthetic with adrenaline at the site of the skin incision further contributes to vasoconstriction and haemostasis, but is not essential in general anaesthetic cases.

Apart from vasoconstriction, several factors help to reduce or control perioperative haemorrhage. Controlled hypotension during general anaesthesia greatly facilitates the surgery and significant bleeding is unusual with a systolic blood pressure below 90mmHg. A head up tilt also reduces cephalic venous pressure and is helpful during both general and local anaesthetic cases. The continuous use of a sucker in the non-dominant hand is a mainstay to aiding viewing, and to displacing tissues and protecting them from other instruments. The appropriate use of bipolar diathermy, careful handling and retraction of the tissues, respect for the surgical planes, and widespread suturing of mucosal flaps, also help to control haemorrhage during open lacrimal surgery. The judicious use of bone wax may, rarely, be necessary to stop persistent haemorrhage from bone.

Surgical technique

A 12–15mm straight skin incision (8–10mm in children), starting just above the medial canthus and extending inferiorly, is made just medial and parallel to the angular vein (Figure 15.1). A straight incision in the thick paranasal skin tends to heal rapidly with an imperceptible scar, whereas more posterior incisions in the concavity of the thinner eyelid skin sometimes heal with a contracted, bridging scar (Figure 15.2). The incision should involve only skin and should not be carried straight down to the bone, as marked haemorrhage is common with the latter approach, due to disruption of the orbicularis muscle and the angular vessels.

The skin is bluntly dissected from the underlying orbicularis oculi muscle, using blunt-tipped scissors directed posteriorly, and the pretarsal and preseptal parts of the orbicularis muscle separated along the line of the fibres down to the bone of the lacrimal crest, using scissors in a spreading motion just lateral to the angular vein. A squint hook is used to retract the preseptal orbicularis and angular vessels medially and any bleeding vessels are carefully cauterised.

A Rollet's rougine is used in an oblique, spreading mode to incise the periosteum on the anterior lacrimal crest, starting at the inferior edge of the medial canthal tendon and

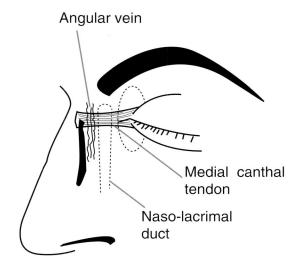

Figure 15.1 Incision for external dacryocysto-rhinostomy (bold line), just medial to the angular vein; the position relative to the medial canthal tendon and lacrimal system (dotted line) is indicated.

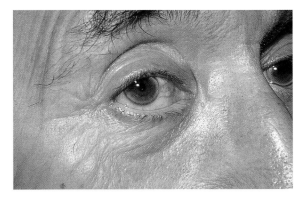

Figure 15.2 Bowed scar due to contracture in a posteriorly-placed dacryocystorhinostomy incision.

extending to the origin of the nasolacrimal duct. Using the sharp cutting edge of the Rollet's rougine, the medial canthal tendon is transected close to its insertion, the periosteum divided up to the top of the lacrimal sac fossa and the paranasal periosteum reflected as far anteriorly as possible. The sucker is used to displace the lacrimal sac laterally, with its periosteal covering, as the periosteum is stripped backwards as far as the posterior lacrimal

crest. At this stage 2/0 silk traction sutures may be passed through the anterior periosteal edge, with encirclement of the orbicularis muscle and angular vessels, and the sutures clipped under tension to the surgical drapes. Similar sutures are used to encircle the orbicularis laterally, the increased surgical exposure and haemostasis being particularly useful for the less-experienced surgeon (Figure 15.3). With local anaesthesia, traction sutures are not possible and a small, self-retaining retractor is a useful alternative.

Having exposed the whole lacrimal sac fossa, the pack or cotton-tipped applicators are removed from the nasal space and the thin bone at the suture between the lacrimal bone and the frontal process of the maxilla is breached with a Traquaire's periosteal elevator. In cases where the bone is extremely thick, a curved haemostat may be required to make the initial break or, failing that, a hammer and chisel may be used to thin the anterior lacrimal crest until the bone can be breached. Some surgeons prefer to use a burr or trephine.

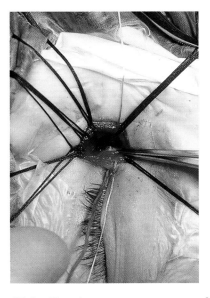

Figure 15.3 Traction sutures are useful for increasing exposure of the operative site, especially for the surgeon in training.

A large rhinostomy is fashioned using bone punches, trephine or a burr. When using punches, it is easiest to first enlarge the opening to at least 1cm in front of the anterior lacrimal crest, as far superiorly as possible; the Traquaire's periosteal elevator being used in a sweeping motion, between bites, to separate the underlying nasal mucosa from the bone. The mucosa is more adherent and more friable anteriorly, where greater care is required. Bone removal from the side of the nose, anterior to the frontal process of the maxilla, is directed inferiorly to about the level of the orbital floor – thereby creating an L-shaped rhinostomy (Figure 15.4); in so doing, the thick bone of the anterior lacrimal crest is significantly weakened and removed relatively easily with a downward-cutting bone punch. The thin bone lying between the upper part of the nasolacrimal duct and the nasal mucosa, the hamular process of the lacrimal bone, is then removed using a Jensen bone nibbler. Attention is now directed superiorly, where further bone should be carefully removed to extend the rhinostomy to the skull base; this is essential to ensure that the internal opening of the common canaliculus is not obstructed by bone or scarring after surgery. Excessive tearing forces should be avoided during bone removal from the upper part of the rhinostomy, as this may very rarely result in a hairline fracture of the cribriform plate and cerebrospinal fluid leak. The rhinostomy should extend posteriorly into the anterior ethmoid air cells, where it is generally necessary to remove small flakes of ethmoid bone to allow an adequate mucosal anastomosis.

Having completed the rhinostomy, a "00" Bowman lacrimal probe is passed via the inferior canaliculus into the lacrimal sac. The probe tents the medial wall of the sac (Figure 15.5), which is then incised using a No. 11 style blade, directed away from the internal opening of the common canaliculus to avoid damaging it. The sac must be widely

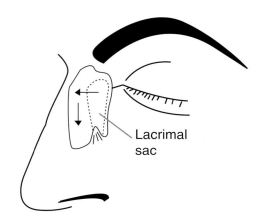

Figure 15.4   Creating the rhinostomy: the arrows indicate the easiest direction of bone removal, relative to the lacrimal sac (dotted line).

opened from the fundus down into the nasolacrimal duct using Westcott scissors or Werb's angled scissors and a common error is to open the relatively thick overlying fascia only, leaving the very thin sac mucosa intact. The lumen of the sac should be examined and the free patency of the internal opening of the common canaliculus confirmed; if the opening is obstructed by a membrane, the obstruction should be carefully excised, using Westcott scissors or a No. 11 blade, and silicone intubation placed.

Being careful to avoid damage to the nasal septum, the nasal mucosa is incised with a

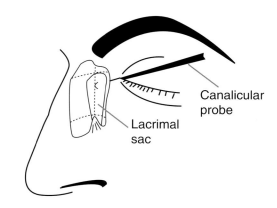

Figure 15.5   Creating mucosal flaps: the canalicular probe tents the medial wall of the lacrimal sac and the dotted lines indicate incisions in the lacrimal sac and nasal mucosa.

No. 11 blade to create a larger anterior flap (about two-thirds of the antero-posterior extent) and a smaller posterior flap and, after cauterisation wherever possible, relieving incisions are made at the superior and inferior bone edges to mobilise both flaps. Incising the nasal mucosa often results in some bleeding which, under general anaesthesia, can be controlled by passing the sucker up the nose and positioning it just behind the posterior flap – thus acting similarly to the second, intranasal "sump" drain placed during surgery under local anaesthesia. A 6/0 absorbable suture on an 8mm diameter half-circle needle is passed through the middle of the free edge of the anterior nasal flap and the ends secured with a bulldog clip, with the needle left attached. This is slung across the nasal bridge to retract the anterior flap medially whilst suturing the posterior flaps (Figure 15.6).

The posterior mucosal flaps are approximated and sutured using a similar 6/0 absorbable suture, the needle being reverse-mounted in an angled, non-locking needle holder in such a way that its entire length is used – this facilitating maximum suture rotation at quite a distance below the small incision. Either a locked continuous suture, or three or four interrupted sutures, is placed from the sac to the nasal mucosa. Keeping the

lacrimal probe in the sac helps to identify and protect the internal opening while the mucosal flaps are being united, and this can later be replaced by intubation where there is common canalicular disease or a markedly inflamed lacrimal sac. The absorbable suture retracting the anterior nasal flap is then used to unite the anterior mucosal flaps and three or four sutures are usually necessary to secure a good anastomosis (Figure 15.7). The cut medial canthal tendon is sutured to the medial periosteum using the same suture, and closure of the orbicularis is not usually necessary if the fibres were bluntly separated in the plane between the palpebral and orbital parts. Skin closure is achieved with 6/0 nylon interrupted or continuous mattress sutures, antibiotic ointment instilled into the conjunctival sac, and a pressure dressing applied to the incision. Post operative haemorrhage is infrequent with primary anastomosis of the mucosal edges, and packing of the nasal space is not required routinely, but an adrenaline-moistened pack may be placed if there is persistent brisk haemorrhage after surgery is completed; such a pack should be left undisturbed for five days.

Post operative management

In the immediate post operative period the patient is nursed semi-erect on bed rest to

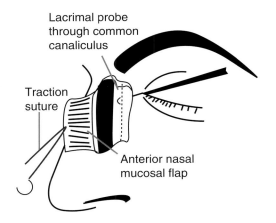

Figure 15.6 Anastomosis of the posterior mucosal flaps, with the anterior nasal mucosal flap held aside by a traction suture resting across the nasal bridge.

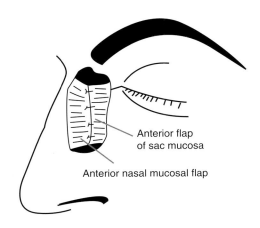

Figure 15.7 Closure of the anterior mucosal flaps.

165

reduce the nasal venous congestion that can contribute to nasal oozing and, for similar reasons, hot drinks should be avoided for 24 hours. A topical combined antibiotic and anti-inflammatory medication is prescribed for a few weeks and, unless systemic antibiotics have been given during surgery, a short course of oral antibiotics is recommended to reduce the incidence of post operative infection. The pressure dressing is removed on the first post operative day and nose blowing discouraged for the first week, to reduce the risk of secondary epistaxis or subcutaneous emphysema. Skin sutures are removed at about one week after surgery and the intubation at about four weeks after surgery, by which time epithelialisation of the surgical fistula has been completed.

Box 15.1 Complications of external lacrimal surgery

Peri-operative
- Canalicular damage
- Haemorrhage
- Cerebrospinal fluid leak
- Inadvertent orbital entry

Post operative
- Haemorrhage
- Wound infection
- Wound necrosis
- Preseptal/orbital cellulitis
- Hypertrophic scar
- Lacrimal tube prolapse
- Medial migration (cheesewiring) of lacrimal tubes

Complications

Serious complications due to external lacrimal surgery are extremely rare, but there are several minor complications (Box 15.1).

In cases of severe continued haemorrhage, nasal packing may be required either with ribbon gauze moistened with a mixture of 1:1000 adrenaline and antibiotics, with an absorbable haemostatic sponge, or with a commercially available expanding nasal tampon.

Minor leak of cerebrospinal fluid may, extremely rarely, result from an inadvertent fracture of the cribriform plate. Once identified, the site of leakage may be plugged with a slip of orbicularis oculi muscle obtained from the surgical field, and post operative systemic antibiotics administered. Although most cases resolve without further complication, close post operative monitoring is required for continued CSF rhinorrhoea or meningitis and neurosurgical advice is recommended.

Orbital fat prolapse may occur if the lateral wall of the lacrimal sac or the orbital periosteum is breached while incising the lacrimal sac or performing a membranectomy. To avoid the risk of orbital haemorrhage, traction on the orbital fat should be avoided in such cases, but a small fat prolapse does not require any specific treatment.

Whilst early post operative nasal oozing is common and requires no treatment except upright positioning of the patient and avoidance of hot beverages, continued brisk primary haemorrhage is very rare. If simple measures, such as pinching of the nasal bridge or icepacks applied to the nasal bridge, do not control brisk primary haemorrhage, then the nose should be packed with 12·5mm ribbon gauze moistened in 1:1000 adrenaline, the pack being left undisturbed for five to seven days and a systemic antibiotic given for that period.

Prophylactic systemic antibiotics reduce the risk of post operative infection (Figure 15.8) and probably reduce the risk of surgical failure. A single dose of a systemic antibiotic is as effective as a post operative course, but antibiotics should be continued after surgery where there has been significant preoperative infection, placement of a nasal tamponade, or significant primary or secondary epistaxis. Use of nasal packs also increases the risk of post operative infection.

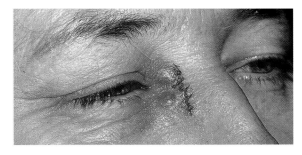

Figure 15.8 Early post operative infective cellulitis around the dacryocystorhinostomy site.

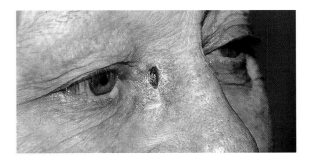

Figure 15.9 Post operative skin necrosis at the dacryocystorhinostomy incision in a patient with previous radiotherapy.

Although the incision line after almost all external DCR is imperceptible by six months, the incision may rarely heal with excessive scar contracture, especially with posteriorly sited incisions (Figure 15.2). Subcutaneous sutures may also increase the tendency to hypertrophic scar formation. Prominent scars may become less noticeable as they mature, especially if massaged or if pressure is applied by, for example, the wearing of glasses on the scar. Very rarely revision of an operative scar is required for unacceptably tight scars, and generally involves a double Z-plasty technique. Wound necrosis is occasionally seen at the incision margins after prior radiotherapy or in patients with Wegener's granulomatosis (Figure 15.9).

Summary

External DCR surgery is a safe and effective procedure for managing troublesome epiphora.

With attention to patient preparation, meticulous surgical technique, an appreciation of the surgical anatomy and careful tissue handling, the surgery should not be unduly difficult and success rates are unmatched by other techniques. For patients without canalicular or lid abnormalities, the "volume" symptoms (due to retention of fluid within the lacrimal sac) can be cured in everybody, whereas "flow" symptoms (due to the tear line height) are affected by canalicular conductance and these symptoms will be improved in at least 95% of cases. Failure is usually due to inadequate primary rhinostomy, failure to create a primary epithelial anastomosis, excessive fibrosis at the rhinostomy site (due to secondary intention healing), stenosis of the canalicular system, or lid abnormalities.

Further reading

Dresner SC, Klussman KG, Meyer DR, Linberg JV. Outpatient dacryocystorhinostomy. *Ophthalmic Surg* 1991; **22**:222–4.

Ezra EJ, Restori M, Mannor GE, Rose GE. Ultrasonic assessment of rhinostomy size following external dacryocystorhinostomy. *Br J Ophthalmology* 1998; **82**:786–9.

Hanna IT, Powrie S, Rose GE. Open lacrimal surgery: a comparison of admission outcome and complications after planned daycase or inpatient management. *Br J Ophthalmol* 1998; **82**:392–6.

Hartikainen J, Grenman R, Pukka P, Seppa H. Prospective randomized comparison of external dacryocystorhinostomy and endonasal laser dacryocystorhinostomy. *Ophthalmology* 1998; **105**:1106–13.

Jordan DR. Avoiding blood loss in outpatient dacryocystorhinostomy. *Ophthal Plast Reconstr Surg* 1991; **7**:261–6.

Jordan DR, Miller D, Anderson RL. Wound necrosis following dacryocystorhinostomy in patients with Wegener's granulomatosis. *Ophthalmic Surg* 1987; **18**:800–3.

Linberg JV. *Lacrimal surgery; contemporary issues in ophthalmology volume 5.* New York: Churchill Livingstone, 1988.

McNab AA. Diagnosis and investigation of lacrimal disease. In McNab AA. *Manual of orbital and lacrimal surgery* (2nd ed.) Oxford: Butterworth Heinemann, 1988.

Neuhaus RW, Baylis HI. Cerebrospinal fluid leakage after dacryocystorhinostomy. *Ophthalmology* 1983; **90**:1091–5.

Tarbet KJ, Custer PL. External dacryocystorhinostomy. Surgical success, patient satisfaction, and economic cost. *Ophthalmology* 1995; **102**:1065–70.

Walland MJ, Rose GE. Soft tissue infections after open lacrimal surgery. *Ophthalmology* 1994; **101**:608–11.

16 Laser-assisted and endonasal lacrimal surgery

Jane M Olver

Endonasal dacryocystorhinostomy is performed entirely within the nose, either by direct visualisation or by using a rigid Hopkins endoscope as the light source and to magnify the structures on the lateral nasal wall. Surgical instruments or laser (or a combination) are used to create an anastomosis between the lacrimal sac and the nasal space (Figure 16.1).

It differs from external DCR (Chapter 15) in that there is no external incision, there are no sutured mucosal flaps and there is usually temporary silicone intubation.

Caldwell, in 1893, first described the use of an electric drill to open the lacrimal sac and nasolacrimal duct into the nasal space from an intranasal approach and West subsequently described another endonasal approach, a so-called "window resection of the nasolacrimal duct". Recognising that the sac-duct junction appeared to be the commonest site of lacrimal outflow obstruction, West later extended the resection to include the lacrimal sac and this remains the principle of modern endonasal lacrimal drainage surgery. Between 1950 and 1990 most lacrimal surgery was performed using an external approach by ophthalmologists, with only few otolaryngologists continuing to practise endonasal surgery. The increased usage of rigid nasal endoscopy and laser surgery has, however, helped to popularise modern endonasal dacryocystorhinostomy, with the results of endonasal endoscopic DCR ranging from 63–99% (Tables 16.1–16.2).

Indications

Endonasal endoscopic DCR is moderately quick, easily performed under local anaesthesia, and bilateral surgery may be

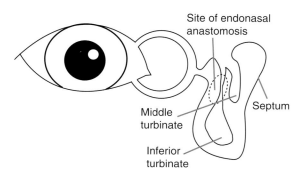

Figure 16.1   Right lacrimal system, with the site of the anastomosis outlined.

Table 16.1   Reported results for endonasal endoscopic surgical dacryocystorhinostomy.

Author	Bone instruments	Number of cases	Success
Whittet	Drill, hammer, chisel, rongeurs	19	94·7%
Weidenbecher	Chisel, drill, backbiting forceps	54	86–95%
Sprekelsen	Drill, rongeur	152	85·5–96%
Yung	Rongeur	81	93%
Zilelioglu	Drill	23	78·3%
Zilelioglu	Drill and Mitomycin C application	14	78·5%
Moore	Chisel, rongeur	34	83%

Table 16.2 Reported results for endonasal laser-assisted dacryocystorhinostomy.

Author	Bone instruments	Number of cases	Success
Gonnering	CO_2 (5) or KTP (15) laser	5 + 15	indeterminate
Woog	Holmium: YAG laser with or without surgical instruments (25 cases where only laser used)	40	82% (72%)
Boush	Argon and surgical instruments	46	70%
Sadiq	Laser (22 cases where no tubes used)	28	79% (59%)
Hartikainen	CO_2 or Nd: YAG	32	63%
Szubin	Argon or Holmium: YAG with surgical instruments	31	97%
Camera	Holmium: YAG laser only	48	89·6%
	Laser with Mitomycin C	123	99·2%

readily performed with relatively little perioperative bleeding. The procedure is, therefore, particularly useful in elderly or frail patients, and in patients who do not wish to accept the low risk of a visible cutaneous scar after external DCR, albeit accepting the higher failure rate for endonasal surgery.

Most cases of primary acquired stenosis, "functional block" or complete obstruction of the nasolacrimal duct are suitable for endonasal DCR, although patients with secondary obstruction may be treated if nasal access is adequate and there is no major nasal disruption. Major mid-facial fractures, being associated with gross disruption of anatomy, are not suitable for this approach and patients with inflammatory nasal diseases associated with scarring (such as sarcoidosis or Wegener's granulomatosis) should probably not undergo endonasal surgery, as the technique is dependent on secondary intention healing. Whilst membranous block of the common canaliculus may be treated during endonasal

dacryocystorhinostomy, more extensive common canalicular block or obstruction of the individual canaliculi is better treated by an external technique (Chapter 17).

Endonasal surgery does not allow a full inspection of the lacrimal sac mucosa and external surgery should, therefore, be used if there is suspicion of a tumour, or other problem, within the lacrimal sac. Other relative contraindications to endonasal DCR include a very narrowed nasal space, a small sac and failed previous DCR with extensive fibrosis at the rhinostomy.

Endonasal endoscopic dacryocystorhinostomy

Local anaesthesia is achieved as previously described (Chapter 15), but with particular attention paid to establishing vasoconstriction of the nasal mucosa (Figure 16.2); it is often necessary to directly infiltrate the submucosal space, anterior to the middle turbinate, using lidocaine 2% with 1:80,000 adrenaline. During the procedure localised haemorrhage may be treated with 1:1000 adrenaline solution applied to the bleeding points with neurosurgical patties.

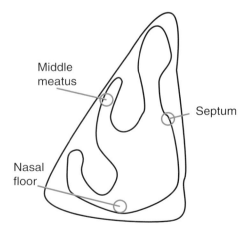

Middle meatus

Septum

Nasal floor

Figure 16.2 Right nasal space; topical anaesthesia and vasoconstrictive medications (both spray and packing) should be applied to these areas before surgery.

Endonasal dacryocystorhinostomy may be performed solely with surgical instrumentation, or with laser-assistance.

Endoscopic surgical dacryocystorhinostomy

After punctal dilation, a 21-gauge vitrectomy light pipe is inserted (unilluminated) into the lacrimal sac, along either canaliculus, and directed infero-medially at an angle of about 40° to the vertical. When illuminated, the light is usually visible on the lateral nasal wall, close to the middle turbinate (Figure 16.3a and 16.3b) and typically anterior to the uncinate process, behind the lacrimal ridge; it may be visible just inside the middle meatus, but sometimes the middle turbinate has to be pushed medially to create adequate operating space. The nasal mucosa overlying the light source is injected with further local anaesthetic.

A flap of nasal mucosa overlying the light source is raised using a Freer elevator (Figure 16.4a and 16.4b) and excised using Blakesley forceps (Figure 16.5a), or the mucosa curetted away with a J-curette, and the thin lacrimal bone pierced and elevated with the Freer elevator and removed with Blakesley forceps (Figure 16.5b). The heavy bone of the frontal process of the maxilla, lying anterior to the area of lacrimal bone removal, should be removed with a Kerrison rongeurs, fine chisel or drill – care being taken not to damage the mucosa of the underlying lacrimal sac or nasolacrimal duct. The light pipe may be used to tent the lacrimal mucosa and feel for residual overlying bone fragments.

The medial wall of the nasolacrimal duct and sac, tented over the light source, is readily opened with an angled keratome and any debris, such as mucopus or dacryoliths, may then be evacuated (Figure 16.6a and 16.6b). Transcanalicular silicone intubation is passed, care being taken not to damage the nasal mucosa whilst withdrawing the bodkins from

the nose, and the ends of the intubation either knotted or clipped together within the nasal space (Figure 16.7a and 16.7b).

Endoscopic laser-assisted dacryocystorhinostomy

Two lasers are in common use for endoscopic laser-assisted dacryocystorhinostomy: the Holmium:YAG (2100nm pulsed) laser is used at 6–8 W for mucosa and 10 W for bone, although the shallow (0·4mm) tissue penetration of this laser is inadequate for removal of the frontal process of the maxilla. The potassium-titanyl-phosphate (KTP) laser, a 532nm superpulsed 15 W laser, is effective for the removal of thicker bone due to good tissue penetration (up to 4mm) and is very well absorbed by haemoglobin, generating excellent haemostasis during surgery.

After local anaesthesia has been induced, the transcanalicular illumination is set-up as for solely surgical endonasal dacryocystorhinostomy. Using a non-contact probe, the laser is used to ablate the nasal mucosa overlying the area of transillumination (Figure 16.8) and, if the laser is of adequate power, the underlying lacrimal bone; all laser-assisted endonasal surgery requires continuous intraoperative aspiration of the smoke plume. It may be necessary to manually remove chips of charred bone from the operative site, and it is often much quicker to remove thick bone (such as the frontal process of the maxilla) using rongeurs. When an adequate rhinostomy has been fashioned, the lacrimal sac and upper duct should be opened with a keratome and silicone intubation placed.

Post operative management and complications

A topical steroid-antibiotic combination should be prescribed and the nose inspected

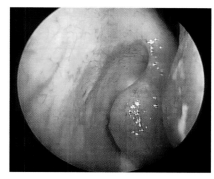

16.3a

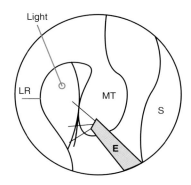

16.3b

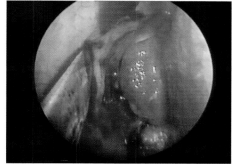

16.4a

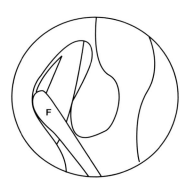

16.4b

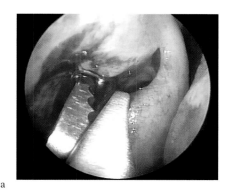

16.5a

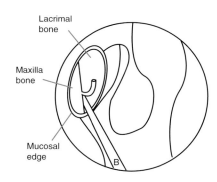

16.5b

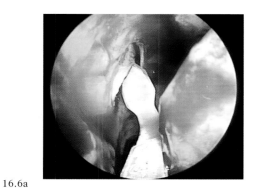

16.6a

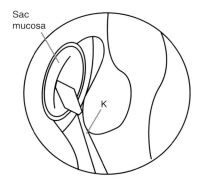

16.6b

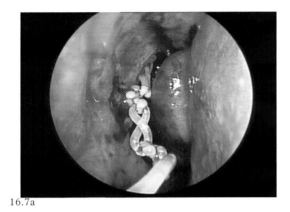

16.7a

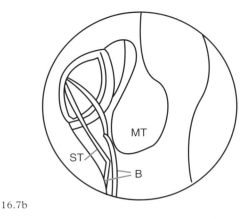

16.7b

Figure 16.3 a–16.7b   Right endonasal surgical DCR:

16.3a The light beam is visible in the middle meatus on the lateral nasal wall; 16.3b view of light-pipe transillumination with 30° Hopkins endoscope, S=septum, LR=lacrimal ridge, MT=middle turbinate, E=endoscope.

16.4a A freer elevator is placed close to the lacrimal ridge, in preparation for raising the mucosal flap (visible blood is from local anaesthesia); 16.4b the mucoperiosteal flap is raised with a freer elevator (F).

16.5a Blakesley forceps are used to grasp and excise nasal mucosa; 16.5b the lacrimal bone is removed with Blakeseley forceps (B).

16.6a The lacrimal sac mucosa is opened with an angled keratome; 16.6b an angled keratome (K) is used to open the lacrimal sac.

16.7a Silicon intubation is passed and knotted in the nasal space; 16.7b the intubation is retrieved from the nose using curved artery forceps, ST=Silicone tube, B=bodkin.

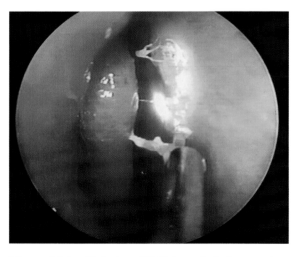

Figure 16.8   Holmium-YAG laser is being used to ablate nasal mucosa, just anterior to the area of transillumination, during left endonasal laser DCR.

in the post operative period. The silicone intubation is typically removed after 6–12 weeks and the function of the anastomosis assessed at about six months.

Complications specific to endonasal surgery may include canalicular damage as a result of the greater instrumentation, collateral laser damage to the mucosa of the nose or lacrimal sac, or the formation of granulation tissue at the rhinostomy or scarring during the healing phase. If the rhinostomy fails due to fibrosis, the anastomosis may be revised either with further endonasal surgery or by external DCR (Chapter 15).

Various success rates have been reported (Tables 16.1 and 16.2), but the perioperative use of a topical anti-metabolite, such as Mitomycin C, appears to reduce the failure rate by decreasing the fibrosis associated with secondary intention healing.

Further reading

Boush GA, Lempke BN, Dortzbach RK. Results of endonasal laser-assisted dacryocystorhinostomy. *Ophthalmology* 1994; **101**:955–9.

Caldwell GW. Two new operations for obstruction of the nasal duct with preservation of the canaliculi, and an incidental description of a new lacrymal probe. *Am J Ophthalmol* 1993; **10**:189–95.

Camera JG, Bennzon AU, Henson RD. The safety and efficacy of mitomycin C in endonasal endoscopic laser-assisted dacryocystorhinostomy. *Ophthal Plast Reconstr Surg* 2000; **16**:114–18.

Gonnering RS, Lyon DB, Fisher JC. Endoscopic laser-assisted lacrimal surgery. *Am J Ophthalmol* 1991; **111**:152–7.

Hartikainen J, Grenman R, Puukka P, Seppa H. Prospective randomised comparison of external dacryocystorhinostomy and endonasal laser dacryocystorhinostomy. *Ophthalmology* 1998; **105**:1106–13.

Jokinen K, Karja J. Endonasal dacryocystorhinostomy. *Arch Otolaryngol* 1974; **100**:41–4.

Massaro BM, Gonnering RS, Harris GJ. Endonasal laser dacryocystorhinostomy. A new approach to nasolacrimal duct obstruction. *Arch Ophthalmol* 1990; **108**:1172–6.

McDonough M, Meiring JH. Endoscopic transnasal dacryocystorhinostomy. *J Laryngol Otol* 1989; **103**:585–7.

Metson R. The endoscopic approach for revision dacryocystorhinostomy. *Laryngoscope* 1990; **100**:1344–7.

Orcutt JC, Hillel A, Weymuller EA. Endoscopic repair of failed dacryocystorhinostomy. *Ophthal Plast Recontr Surg* 1990; **6**:197–202.

Rouviere P, Vaille G, Garcia C, Teppa H, Freche C, Lerault P. La dacryocysto-rhinostomie par voie endo-nasale. *Ann Otolaryngol Chir Cervicofac* 1981; **98**:49–53.

Sadiq SA, Hugkulstone CE, Jones NSS, Downes RN. Endoscopic holmium:YAG laser dacryocystorhinostomy. *Eye* 1996; **10**:43–6.

Sprekelsen MB, Barberan MT. Endoscopic dacryo-cystorhinostomy: surgical technique and results. *Laryngoscope* 1996; **106**:187–9.

Steadman MG. Transnasal dacryocystorhinostomy. *Otolaryngol Clin North Am* 1985; **18**:107–11.

Szubin L, Papageorge A, Sacks E. Endonasal laser assisted dacryocystorhinostomy. *Am J Rhinol* 1999; **13**:371–4.

Weidenbecher M, Hoseman W, Buhr W. Endoscopic endonasal dacryocystorhinostomy: results in 56 patients. *Ann Otol Rhino Laryngol* 1994; **103**:363–7.

West JM. A window resection of the nasal duct in cases of stenosis. *Trans Am Ophthalmol Soc* 1909-11; **12**:654–8.

West JM. The intranasal lacrimal sac operation. Its advantages and its results. *Arch Ophthalmol* 1926; **56**:351–6.

Whittet HB, Shun-Shin GA, Awdry P. Functional endoscopic transnasal dacryocystorhinostomy. *Eye* 1993; 7:545–9.

Woog JJ, Metson R, Puliafito CA. Holmium:YAG endonasal laser dacryocystorhinostomy. *Am J Ophthalmol* 1993; **116**:1–10.

Yung MW, Hardman-Lea S. Endoscopic inferior dacryocystorhinostomy. *Clin Otolaryngol* 1998, **23**:152–7.

Zilelioglu G, Ugurbas SH, Anadolu Y, Akiner M, Akturk T. Adjunctive use of Mitomycin C on endoscopic lacrimal surgery. *Br J Ophthalmol* 1998; **82**:63–6.

17 Specialist lacrimal surgery and trauma

Alan A McNab

Lacrimal canalicular obstruction presents a difficult area for assessment and treatment and the management of traumatic telecanthus and canthal dystopia also falls within this setting. The management of acute lacrimal trauma, including canalicular lacerations, is covered in Chapter 2.

Assessment

The assessment of the lacrimal system is similar to that for more simple lacrimal disorders (Chapter 15) but, in addition, a more extensive assessment of the eye, eyelids, medial canthus and lacrimal system is essential to establish a plan of management. In addition, the nasal structure and cavity should also be carefully examined.

Lacrimal canalicular obstructions may rarely be idiopathic, but are generally the result of infection (primary Herpes simplex and zoster, or Actinomyces canaliculitis), trauma (direct, iatrogenic or irradiation), cicatrising mucous membrane diseases (pemphigoid, chronic ocular medication, or topical drug reactions such as Stevens-Johnson syndrome), or involvement with tumours (papillomas or secondary to skin tumours). With these causes in mind, associated abnormalities should be sought during the ocular examination; for example, in the presence of a progressive disease such as ocular pemphigoid, it may be undesirable to place a canalicular bypass tube for fear of exacerbating inner canthal scarring or worsening an underlying dry eye syndrome.

The shape and position of the medial canthus should be assessed and, if abnormal, the lateral or vertical displacement should be measured relative to the midline and compared with the other side (if normal); the normal adult intercanthal distance is about 30mm, or 15mm from the midline to each canthus. The shape of the canthus may be relevant both for cosmesis and, where required, for the likelihood of being able to successfully place a lacrimal canalicular bypass tube.

Clinical assessment of the lacrimal system is directed towards establishing at what level obstruction lies (Chapter 10). With canalicular obstructions the length of patent canaliculus, both upper and lower, should be measured; the critical length in planning surgery is 8mm. Where there is at least this amount of one remaining canaliculus, it is generally feasible to perform a canaliculo-dacryocystorhinostomy (canaliculo-DCR). If there is less than 8mm, a Lester Jones canalicular bypass tube may be required unless the obstruction lies in the proximal canaliculus; in the latter instance the distal remnants of the canaliculi may be normal and may be opened into the tear lake by retrograde probing from within the lacrimal sac and canaliculostomy, or by direct cut-down along the eyelid margin and intubation of the openings. Although such procedures may be performed without dacryocystorhinostomy, it is more logical to perform DCR at the time of primary canalicular surgery. DCR not only increases canalicular conductance by having bypassed the physiological resistance of the nasolacrimal duct, but adequate primary rhinostomy allows the relatively straight-forward closed placement of a canalicular bypass tube should the primary canalicular surgery fail to control symptoms.

Where there is blockage of each individual canaliculus, the length of patent canaliculus can be estimated clinically and dacryocystography is not possible. With common canalicular obstruction, where syringing leads to reflux of dye-free fluid from the opposite punctum (Chapter 10), a dacryocystogram is helpful in establishing the extent of common canalicular disease. Lateral obstruction, with complete obliteration of the common canaliculus, requires canaliculo-DCR whereas medial obstruction, due to adherence and fibrosis of the mucosal valve over the common canalicular opening, may be dealt with by excision of the membrane at the time of DCR and intubation.

There is no need for CT of the facial skeleton when considering lacrimal surgery after previous mid-facial trauma, provided that the presence of a nasal space alongside the site of future rhinostomy is established by clinical inspection or nasal endoscopy. Where there has been major facial trauma, however, CT of this region may be useful in case other procedures – such as septoplasty, sinus surgery or intercanthal wiring – are to be combined with the lacrimal reconstruction.

Surgical options

Canaliculo-dacryocystorhinostomy (CDCR)

Canaliculo-dacryocystorhinostomy is indicated where there is bicanalicular block with canalicular obstruction situated a minimum of 8mm from at least one of the puncta and for *lateral* common canalicular block, in which several millimetres of common canaliculus have been obliterated by scar tissue. The principle of the procedure is to excise the block of scar tissue and unite the medial end of one or both canaliculi to the nose, using the lacrimal sac mucosa as a bridging flap; the operation, although technically feasible, carries a much lower success rate than the standard external DCR or surgery for a more medial common canalicular obstruction (Chapter 15) and closed placement of a Lester Jones canalicular bypass tube may be required later if the operation fails.

A standard DCR incision is made but, before mobilising the lacrimal sac and periosteum, probes are placed in the blocked canaliculi, and the overlying medial canthal tendon divided and dissected laterally using blunt or sharp dissection (Figure 17.1a). This dissection is continued laterally until the tips of the canalicular probes are revealed in the underlying tissues, the ends of the canaliculi are transected at their most medial point and fine silicone tubing inserted and pulled laterally, to aid in retraction. If only one canaliculus is patent, either a monocanalicular stent can be used, or the other end of a bicanalicular intubation can be returned to the nasal space through a "blind" passage (via the punctal annulus, if present), ensuring entry into the nasal space well away from the one remaining functional canaliculus.

A large rhinostomy is created and nasal mucosal flaps fashioned (Figure 17.1b); with canaliculo-DCR, however, a very large anterior nasal flap is required and relatively small posterior flap. The lacrimal sac is opened, not in the mid-part of its medial wall – as with ordinary DCR (Chapter 15) – but much more anteriorly at the junction of the medial wall and anterior border; this allows the lacrimal sac to be "unfurled" posteriorly to create a large bridging flap between the back wall of the canaliculi and the small posterior nasal flap. The canalicular mucosa is united to the small anterior edge of

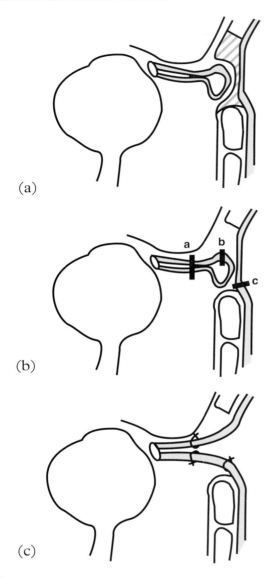

(a)

(b)

(c)

Figure 17.1 Representation of canaliculo-dacryocystorhinostomy:
(a) The lacrimal sac in its fossa with an obstruction of the distal canaliculus and the area of bone removal for the rhinostomy (hatched).
(b) The sites of incision marked: "a" denotes an incision across the most medial portion of the patent canaliculus, "b" the incision in the anterior aspect of the lacrimal sac and "c" the incision in the nasal mucosa to make a large anterior mucosal flap and a small posterior flap.
(c) The anastomosis performed with the anterior nasal mucosal flap sutured to the canaliculus and the lacrimal sac opened out and sutured as a "bridging flap" between the nasal mucosa and the posterior edge of the lacrimal canaliculi.

the lacrimal sac mucosa with two or three 8/0 absorbable sutures and the posterior edge of the sac sutured to the nasal mucosa using 6/0 absorbable sutures. The canalicular intubation is knotted as with a standard DCR, passed into the nasal space and the anterior mucosal anastomosis between the large nasal flap and the anterior edge of the canalicular remnants completed with multiple 8/0 absorbable sutures (Figure 17.1c); it is important to avoid snagging the intubation with the cutting edge of the needles whilst performing the anterior mucosal union. Finally the DCR wound is closed in a standard fashion and the intubation left in place for several months. If watering continues at 9–12 months after canaliculo-DCR, closed placement of a Lester Jones canalicular bypass tube is required.

Complications

Although canaliculo-DCR has the same spectrum of complications as simple DCR (Chapter 15), the commonest specific complication is failure of tear drainage due to re-obstruction of the fine surgical anastomosis. Trephination and silicone intubation may be tried where the obstruction is a small membrane, but in most cases the closed placement of a Lester Jones bypass tube will required.

Dacryocystorhinostomy with retrograde canaliculostomy

Indications

This procedure is designed to open onto the lid margin, in the region of the medial tear lake, canaliculi that are blocked within their first 6–7mm but are patent in the distal part; it being, of course, only possible to establish this at the time of surgery and so the patient must be warned that a glass canalicular bypass tube might be required if there is insufficient canaliculus to allow a retrograde canaliculostomy.

A standard external DCR is performed to the point of opening the lacrimal sac and suturing of the posterior mucosal flaps (Chapter 15). The common canalicular opening is located in the usual fashion and a "0" gauge lacrimal probe, bent perpendicularly on itself at about 8–10mm from the end, is then passed from the sac, into the common canaliculus (Figure 17.2a) and as far laterally as possible along each canaliculus. The probe is pushed up against the lid margin and a cut down made onto the end of the probe, opening the canaliculus onto the lid margin (Figure17.2b) and the same manoeuvre repeated for the other canaliculus, if possible. The "false" puncta are intubated and the DCR completed in a standard fashion; if only one canaliculus is present, the other end of the intubation is returned to the nasal space through a "blind" passage. A monocanalicular stent placed in the pseudo-punctum is unlikely to remain in position in the absence of the normal punctal annulus.

The intubation can be removed when the epithelium of the canaliculus and the conjunctiva have united and there is little need to leave them more than 3–4 weeks, or the tubes will tend to "cheese wire" through the tissues and cause a medial cross-union between the eyelids. If the pseudo-puncta fail to control symptoms, closed placement of a canalicular bypass tube is required.

Dacryocystorhinostomy and Jones canalicular bypass tube

The canalicular bypass tube is designed to establish tear drainage, from the medial tear lake into the nose, by way of a false conduit; the most used device being the Pyrex glass (Lester Jones) canalicular bypass tube. Placement of a bypass tube is indicated where the extent of canalicular obliteration is such as to preclude either canaliculo-DCR or DCR with retrograde canaliculostomy, or where watering continues in the face of a functioning

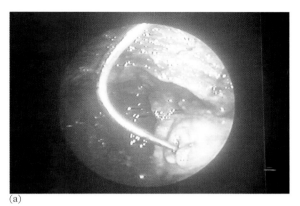
(a)

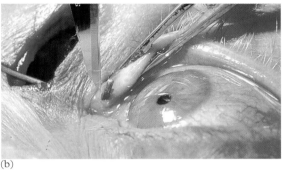
(b)

Figure 17.2 Retrograde canaliculostomy during dacryocystorhinostomy: (a) the angled "0" gauge probe is being directed towards the internal opening of the common canaliculus in the left lacrimal sac; (b) a cut-down on the lid margin is directed onto the most lateral point reached by the probe placed retrogradely into the canaliculus.

standard DCR – as, for example, in patients with facial nerve palsy.

As with DCR and retrograde canaliculostomy, a standard external DCR is performed to the stage of suturing the posterior mucosal flaps although, if no lacrimal sac is present or flaps cannot be formed, the posterior nasal mucosa should be sutured to the soft tissues of the lacrimal sac fossa. Although a large rhinostomy is important for all lacrimal surgery (Chapter 15), it is particularly important when placing a canalicular bypass tube, or the tube tends to become displaced due to its bearing on the bone at the lower edge of the rhinostomy. The nasal cavity should also be examined and, if necessary, the anterior part of the middle turbinate should be de-boned or trimmed to make extra room for the medial end of the tube.

If retrograde exploration of the common canaliculus fails to reveal any useful tissues for retrograde canaliculostomy, a carunculectomy may be performed with care being taken to avoid damage to the plica semilunaris. A sharp guide wire is inserted from the medial canthus into the nose (Figure 17.3). The point of entry is critical to the functional success of the tube and should be at the level of the undisplaced lower eyelid margin, at the site of carunculectomy. An alternative site is the lateral 2–3mm of the canaliculus which, if present, can be laid open to accommodate the lateral flanged end of the bypass tube. The wire marks the future track of the tube and is directed about 15–25° downhill in the coronal plane, the medial end passing into the nose in the vicinity of the lacrimal sac fossa.

A small trephine (1·5–2mm diameter) is passed over the guide wire to remove a narrow core of tissue and, whilst the trephine is in the tissues, the sharp wire may be replaced with a blunt one. A glass canalicular bypass tube is slipped over the guide wire and pushed firmly through the tissues so that the distal end is at least 2mm clear within the nasal space; the end of a thumb-nail should be used to drive the tube into the tissues, as instruments tend to shatter the glass flange of the tube. The neck of the tube is encircled with three turns of a 6/0 nylon suture, passed through the medial end of the lower lid and tied over the bolster – this suture lifting the tube slightly laterally to allow epithelial healing around (and not over) the lateral end of the bypass tube. In most cases a 12mm tube with a 3·5mm flange is suitable for caruncular placement, whereas a somewhat longer (16mm) tube may be needed where the neck of the bypass tube is placed within the lateral canalicular remnant.

The anterior mucosal anastomosis and surface closure is completed as with standard external DCR. The encircling suture is

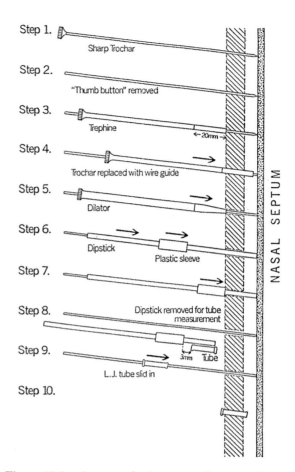

Figure 17.3   A system for insertion of a Lester Jones bypass tube using a guide wire, trephine and "dipstick". (Reproduced with permission from Morlet GC. A modern approach to lacrimal surgery. *Aust NZ J Ophthalmol* 1988; **16**:202.)

removed at 7–10 days after surgery, at the time of suture removal from the skin incision.

Canalicular bypass tubes are subject to a number of common complications and require regular monitoring and maintenance, otherwise they become caked or blocked with mucus debris from the tear film and this results in recurrent conjunctivitis. Patients should be encouraged to sniff water from the tear lake, through the tube and into the nose, on a daily basis and they should also be taught to place one of their fingers over the tube when violently sneezing or nose blowing.

Lateral migration of the tube occurs most often and the tube will sometimes be completely dislodged, when closed replacement should be undertaken. Repeated episodes of tube extrusion generally occur due to residual bone in the area of the rhinostomy and, in such cases, open revision of the rhinostomy should be undertaken. More rarely the tube will sink medially into the tissues and may require a cut-down to retrieve it.

Malposition of the ocular end of the tube may result in failure of tear drainage where the tube is too anterior or, more usually, the tube is too posterior and becomes embedded in conjunctiva or against the globe, causing episcleritis. In more extreme cases, the irritation will cause formation of a pyogenic granuloma – this being particularly troublesome where the tube has become filthy through neglect. In such cases of malposition with secondary inflammation, the tube should be removed and replaced in a better position at a later date when the inflammatory changes have settled.

Build-up of tear-film debris on the surface of a bypass tube tends to lead to obstruction and repeated ocular infections. If the obstruction cannot be cleared with the tube in place, the device should be removed and cleaned, or else replaced.

Closed placement of a canalicular bypass tube

Indications

Closed secondary placement of a glass canalicular bypass tube is indicated when a previously inserted bypass tube has become dislodged, after failed canaliculo-DCR or retrograde canaliculostomy, or where, in the absence of reflex lacrimation, a functioning DCR fails to control watering.

The procedure is similar to a primary (open) bypass tube, except that the DCR has already been performed and the rhinostomy does not have to be opened; in other words, the tube is inserted in a closed fashion. For optimum positioning of the distal end of the bypass tube, nasal examination is required and is best achieved with endoscopy, although a good headlight and nasal speculum are often adequate. A 3mm diameter rigid sucker is required to clean the nasal space during surgery. The procedure is best performed under general anaesthesia as vasoconstriction from the endonasal local anaesthesia encourages, due to an artificially shrunken middle turbinate and septal mucosa, a misjudgement of the position of the nasal end of the tube.

First-time placement of a closed Jones' tube is similar to the open canalicular bypass tube, using and positioning the guide wire and trephine in the same way; the intranasal position of the introducer should be checked endoscopically and, if necessary, the anterior part of the middle turbinate removed to make room for the tube. If there has recently been a satisfactorily functioning tube, the double-ended ("bullhorn") dilator that accompanies the commercial sets of tubes may be used to dilate the previous track and the tube forced into place along an "0" gauge probe introduced into the dilated track. After placement of any bypass tube, the position of both the ocular and the nasal ends of the unsupported tube should be checked and it is particularly important to verify that the nasal end lies free within the nasal cavity and not up against the septum, lateral wall or turbinate. A newly-placed tube needs to be secured in the same way as a primary tube, but a replacement tube does not need fixation.

Medial canthoplasty during lacrimal surgery

Where injury to the lacrimal drainage system has been accompanied by significant midfacial trauma, there may be traumatic telecanthus or canthal dystopia and repositioning of the canthus may be required as part of the lacrimal surgical repair. Malpositions of the canthus secondary to trauma are, however, notoriously difficult to correct and, despite the best efforts, the canthus tends to drift back towards its previous position.

Traumatic telecanthus may be due to a widening of the fractured midfacial skeleton and the first step required may be to remove excess bone at the inner canthi, this then presenting difficulty with the medial fixation of the inner canthi in the absence of a firm bony anchor. In this setting a transnasal wire is helpful (Chapter 6) or a small T-plate or anchor-screw – to which to fix the canthal tendon – may be inserted into the remaining fragments of the nasal bones. To facilitate a medial repositioning of the lids, it is important to widely mobilise the medial attachments of the eyelids.

If canthal repositioning is being performed at the time of open lacrimal surgery, advantage can be made of exposure of the posterior lacrimal crest and this fascia used as an anchor point for elevating the medial end of the lower eyelid. Although some results will be encouraging (Figure 17.4), on occasion this site of postero-superior fixation lacks rigidity.

The superficial tissues may need to be redistributed at the time of surgery. In traumatic canthal dystopia, the canthus is generally shifted downwards and a triangular pedicle flap of skin, based medially on the side of the nasion, may be transposed from the upper eyelid to the lower; this thereby helping to raise the inner canthus by correcting any vertical shortage of tissues below the medial canthus (Figure 17.5).

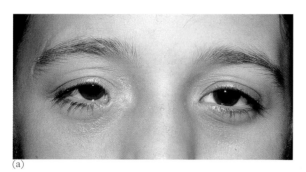
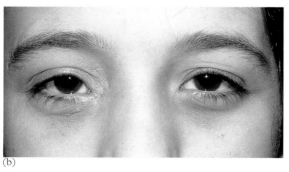

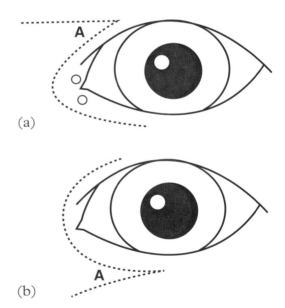

Figure 17.4 Medial canthoplasty performed at the time of open lacrimal surgery: (a) pre- and (b) post surgery. Although there is an improvement in the canthal position and elevation after postero-superior fixation of the lower eyelid, this is limited by scarring at the site of the previous injury.

Figure 17.5 Redistribution of the soft tissues as part of a medial canthoplasty for inferior displacement of the medial canthus. The apex 'A' of the flap of skin and muscle is transposed from the upper eyelid (a) into the lower (b) after fixing the canthal structures deeply to bone or periosteum.

Further reading

Bartley GB, Gustafson RO. Complications of malpositioned Jones tubes. *Am J Ophthalmol* 1990; **109**:66–9.

Call NB, Welham RAN. Epiphora after irradiation of medial eyelid tumors. *Am J Ophthalmol* 1981; **92**:842–5.

Chapman KL, Bartley GB, Garrity JA, Gonnering RS. Lacrimal bypass surgery in patients with sarcoidosis. *Am J Ophthalmol* 1999; **127**:443–6.

Coster DJ, Welham RAN. Herpetic canalicular obstruction. *Br J Ophthalmol* 1979; **63**:259–62.

Henderson ON. A modified trephining technique for insertion of Lester Jones tube. *Arch Ophthalmol* 1985; **103**:1582–5.

Hicks C, Pitts J, Rose GE. Lacrimal surgery in patients with congenital cranial or facial anomalies. *Eye* 1994; **8**:583–91.

Jones BR. The surgical cure of obstruction of the common canaliculus. *Trans Ophthalmol Soc UK* 1960; **80**:343–56.

Kwan ASL, Rose GE. Lacrimal drainage surgery in Wegener's granulomatosis. *Br J Ophthalmol* 2000; **84**:329–31.

McLean CJ, Rose G.E. Post-herpetic lacrimal obstruction. *Ophthalmology* 2000; **107**:496–9.

McNab AA. Lacrimal canalicular obstruction associated with topical ocular medication. *Aust NZ J Ophthalmol* 1998; **26**:219–24.

McNab AA. Diagnosis and investigation of lacrimal disease. In: McNab AA, ed, *Manual of orbital and lacrimal surgery* (2nd ed). Oxford: Butterworth Heinemann, 1988: 91–8.

Morlet GC. A modern approach to lacrimal surgery. *Aust NZ J Ophthalmol* 1988; **16**:199–204.

Rose GE, Welham RAN. Jones' lacrimal canalicular bypass tubes: twenty-five years' experience. *Eye* 1991; **5**:13–19.

Sanke RF, Welham RAN. Lacrimal canalicular obstruction and chicken pox. *Br J Ophthalmol* 1982; **66**:71–4.

Steinsapir KD, Glatt HJ, Putterman AM. A 16-year study of conjunctival dacryocystorhinostomy. *Am J Ophthalmol* 1990; **109**:387–93.

Wearne MJ, Beigi B, Davis G, Rose GE. Retrograde intubation dacryocystorhinostomy for proximal and mid-canalicular obstruction. *Ophthalmology* 1999; **106**:2325–8.

Index

Page numbers in **bold** refer to figures; those in *italic* refer to tables or boxed material

182